Performance Philosophy

Performance Philosophy is an interdisciplinary and international field of thought, creative practice and scholarship. The Performance Philosophy book series comprises monographs and essay collections addressing the relationship between performance and philosophy within a broad range of philosophical traditions and performance practices, including drama, theatre, performance arts, dance, art and music. It also includes studies of the performative aspects of life and, indeed, philosophy itself. As such, the series addresses the philosophy of performance as well as performance-as-philosophy and philosophy-as-performance.

http://www.performancephilosophy.org/books/

More information about this series at
http://www.palgrave.com/gp/series/14558

Eva Schuermann

Seeing as Practice

Philosophical Investigations into the Relation between Sight and Insight

palgrave
macmillan

Eva Schuermann
Otto-von-Guericke University
Magdeburg, Germany

Translated by
Steven Black
Academy of Fine Arts Leipzig
Leipzig, Germany

Performance Philosophy
ISBN 978-3-030-14506-4 ISBN 978-3-030-14507-1 (eBook)
https://doi.org/10.1007/978-3-030-14507-1

Cover illustration: still from the film '*Felix in Exile*', by courtesy of the artist © William Kentridge

This Palgrave Macmillan imprint is published by the registered company Springer Nature Switzerland AG
The registered company address is: Gewerbestrasse 11, 6330 Cham, Switzerland

Contents

Preface to the translated edition 2018

This is a translation of my German book *Sehen als Praxis* originally published by Suhrkamp in 2008. It is not a revised second edition. The text has been delicately edited, but the gist and structure of the argument have been kept as they were. Of course, since its original publication, debates around vision and mind have continued, above all as a result of insights gained from the neurosciences and new techniques of visualisation. Thinking about vision involves questions that pertain to the relation between mind and world, as well as to the relation between mind and brain. I discuss this as the interconnectedness of sight and insight with reference to concrete cases of aesthetical and ethical experiences.

The main theoretical context in which I situate my argument relates to the notion of practice that goes back to the later Wittgenstein. Practice means that seeing is an action situated in contexts, i.e. it is simultaneously determined and determining. With the help of this notion, I hope to provide a persuasive alternative to what the editors of an anthology of philosophy of perception call "the orthodox view" (Thompson and Noë 2002), which regards vision as a functional representation and disregards the fact that it is an action that is socially learned and conditioned.

This focus on practice explains why the book is well placed in the *Performance Philosophy* book series because performativity is the salient feature of each practice. It means that actions are not only individual activities or processes of doing something; rather, they also have executive, embodying qualities that shape social realities. It is by drawing on these concepts that I have sought to find a third way between a constructivist and a representationalist[1] notion of seeing.

The words performativity and performance are, however, notoriously ambiguous and can be quite unclear. They can be used to describe anything from circus spectacles to embodiment practices. My basic idea goes back to Austin (1962) who revealed the performativity of speech acts. Analogously, my claim is that seeing is an act that can be realised very differently, although it is conditioned by the nature of the eye and the seen thing. The way we perceive is thus neither independent of the perceived nor of the perceiver. Rather, it is *how* we look at something that constitutes *what* it *actually* is. As an act of qualitative performance, seeing primarily gives rise to the seen thing.

The performative dimension of seeing, i.e., the way seeing embodies expression, is particularly conspicuous in the act of seeing both persons and art works. The performative is emergent in the sense that it refers not to something already given, but to the procedural nature of what is thereby being created or produced, while at the same time focusing on the aesthetic and responsive qualities at play in that process.

I am grateful to Steven Black, the careful translator, and to Sebastian Spanknebel, Shefika Doghan and Rudolf Müllan for further preparing the manuscript for publication. Many thanks also to William Kentridge's studio for providing the images of his work, and to Levno von Plato for clearing the rights for the other images and for his comments. Finally, I owe special thanks to Alice Lagaay for taking the book into the *Performance Philosophy* series and for supervising the publication process.

References

Austin, John Langshaw. 1962. *How to Do Things with Words: The William James Lectures Delivered at Harvard University in 1955.* Oxford: Clarendon Press.

Thompson, Evan, and Noë, Alva (ed.). 2002. *Introduction. Vision and Mind: Selected Readings in the Philosophy of Perception.* Cambridge: MIT Press.

[1] Under the umbrella term 'representation,' a very heterogenous matter is conceived. Herewith, I refer to the misleading concept of mirroring something in a pre-given form, i.e. simply passively receiving something caused by the seen object that is allegedly just given.

List of Figures

Chapter 4

Chapter 9

CHAPTER 1

Introduction: Why Seeing is a Practice

"The concept of 'seeing' makes a tangled impression. Well, it is tangled." (Ludwig Wittgenstein 1986, 200).

This book investigates the power of vision in terms of its structure and its modes of operation. Everyone sees from an individual perspective, from a unique location in space and in their own particular way. We can nevertheless communicate tolerably well amongst each other concerning what we see. Seeing is both a proven means of orientation, of acquiring information and of interacting with others, and at the same time a personality-specific way of perceiving reality conditioned by individual and cultural variations. Neither modes of seeing can be fully explained by our knowledge of retinal and neuronal processing (physiology) or by empirical Gestalt theory (psychology). In general, a type of constative *seeing that* is regarded as the least problematic instance of epistemic perception, whereas all more complex cases of *seeing something as something* are regarded in terms of interpretative or metaphorical reference to the seen.

Philosophy has been primarily interested in vision as a means of obtaining knowledge, and philosophical approaches have always oscillated between objectivist and subjectivist views. In the former, perception is conceived either as a causally determined representation of the outside world, or simply understood in terms of physiological stimulus response. The latter view characterises the seeing subject as the autonomous constructor of their

E. Schuermann, *Seeing as Practice*, Performance Philosophy,
https://doi.org/10.1007/978-3-030-14507-1_1

own world, thereby removing emphasis from any historically and culturally productive, yet contingent, freedom within seeing. Both versions impose significant restrictions on understanding what seeing could be. The objectivist approach fails to take mediation into account, while the subjectivist approach, in so far as it fails to acknowledge history and culture, is somewhat solipsistic. Too much, and also too little, is asked both of the seeing person and the polyvalent *visible*, i.e. of consciousness and the world. Again, the objectivist interpretation is unable to explain the variations and divergences in individual perception; it does not account for why everyone sees differently, why visible things can be overlooked, and why we always see both more *and* less than what is there to be seen. Similarly, the subjectivist conception cannot plausibly explain the degree of intersubjective convergence between my personal perception and that of others. Although everything physical within a given space is visible physiologically, not everything in such a view is noticed and seen in accord with the way others see it. It follows that seeing is neither perceiving the pure representation of a physically present world, nor the pure construction of an individual viewpoint, although it nevertheless contains aspects of both. To understand vision as simply recognition in terms of replicating reality, the visible as merely objective presence, is to ignore the generative capacity and the relative nature of the faculty of vision.

A philosophical theory of perception needs to engage with the tension at the core of a perceptual world that is both socially shared and private. It also needs to determine the relation between sense and sensibility, sight and insight, seeing and ways of seeing. As an activity of consciousness, seeing is interconnected with other mental acts of representation and judgement, with affective dispositions of hoping, desiring, fearing, as well as with temporal referencing in memory and expectation. This would be difficult to explain if seeing were solely a means of attaining knowledge. A second problem to resolve consists thereby in the relation of perception to thinking and believing, to representation and imagination, to constative and interpretive acts.

A third difficulty is posed by the diversity of forms of seeing. Any attempt to understand seeing must take into account a multiplicity of uses and contexts of use that are peculiar to visual perception. This multiplicity undermines or relativises the paradigm of seeing as recognition and predication, and recasts the form of visual perception par excellence as only one aspect of a set of multiform variations and modalities of perceptual relation to the world: the scientific researcher's gaze, the meaningful speaking gaze and the pensive lost gaze each disclose a particular sphere of the visible. The interpersonal gaze occurs as an event through which the self is mirrored back as it appears to the other.

The relation between the viewer and the visible must consequently be considered within an entirely different interpretive framework. If preconceptions about vision and visibility are indeed presupposed, then seeing is understood as a means of accessing the world that provides knowledge and conclusions about things sensibly present in the world. I want to depart from this preconception to arrive at a more finely nuanced description of what happens when someone sees. Neither empiricist sense data theories nor constructivist theories of vision are sufficient tools in themselves to conceptually grasp the uniquely protean predisposition of the faculty of vision, situated as it is *between* consciousness and world, construction and representation, interpretation and response, state and action. There is good reason to regard seeing as a contextually situated and intersubjective *activity*, i.e. action that engenders or generates something.

1 Two Cases of Perceptual World Disclosure

What parents do when they look at their child with a gaze that conveys the warning: "careful now, don't push it," is an "act" that cannot be described and understood solely in terms of an epistemic or representational notion of perception. Such explanatory schemes are even less appropriate for grasping what the infant does when it *sees* that its parents are angry. By looking at their child, the parents perform illocutionary acts of communication; they do something by seeing. The infant in turn performs, by seeing, an act of sense disclosure. If this occurrence is separated out into sensory impulse reception on the basis of light waves on the one hand, and interpretive attribution of meaning on the other, the result is to obstruct any understanding of it as a meaningful and successful integral act. Epistemic elements may indeed be involved in this type of seeing; for instance, the parents may 'recognise' that their child is behaving badly or the child may have the 'insight' that its parents are offended by something. Nonetheless, this is not simply a case of understanding occasioned by the sense of sight, but rather of meaning accomplished by shared, perceptive world disclosure. The infant is confronted with what it is, literally, *in the eyes* of its parents. The encounter is literal and not metaphorical because it becomes noticeable first and foremost *aisthetically*—that is, sensorially. It involves interpersonal perceptions that the participants have of each other, which prompt them to do what they do—to reprove, to feel bad, to conform or to rebel.

A further example of the multi-layered character of aisthesis is the type of seeing characterised by Petrarch's ascent of Mont Ventoux, in which seeing became an aesthetic perception and end in itself—in Petrarch's case the perception of landscape. Regardless of how constructed this episode of European cultural history may be, no one would have declared Petrarch's journey in 1336 to indicate an epochal turn in the European perception of landscape had his initial act of perception been merely the result of his mirroring re-cognition of an objectively given world.

The main reason his account of the ascent to the summit could lead to philosophical-historical and speculative reconstructions was that it expressed a fundamental change of orientation and offered a new perceptual paradigm. To climb a mountain just "to *see* what so great an elevation had to offer" (Petrarca 1898, p. 308, cursive ES) marks a break with the instrumentalist semantics of seeing. Giving himself over to the contemplation of the landscape, Petrarch's describes his state thus: "owing to the unaccustomed quality of the air and the effect of the great sweep of view spread out before me, I stood like one dazed" (ibid., p. 313). His case exemplifies an important distinction, namely that between seeing for the pleasure and emotion of it and seeing for some ulterior purpose in everyday life.

Petrarch's example also makes it possible to understand how sight and insight, aisthetic and theoretical vision[1] can merge into one another. The poet does not linger long before the sight of the French Alps in the clouds; his enjoyment of the view soon is transformed into theoretical reflection on the divine order of the world. An activity with a purely aesthetic end can in this way develop into philosophical contemplation because observation is a Janus-headed activity directed neither purely outwards nor inwards but instead always involving "parallel actions." The sentience of seeing cannot be separated from its capacity to generate meaning.

Petrarch's sight of the panorama is immediately accompanied by qualms about admiring the terrestrial.[2] After having begun his descent, he writes, "I was satisfied that I had seen enough of the mountain; I turned my inward eye upon myself" (Petrarca 1898, p. 317). He thus provides an excellent example of the seeing subject as at once *bios praktikos and theoretikos*, at

[1] Hans Blumenberg (1973) reads the report in Petrarca's letter as an epochal change in the history of the theoretical exploration of the world.

[2] On this interpretation, see Ritter (1989).

once active and contemplative. The intelligible character of sight—in its more than merely metaphorical proximity to insight and to processes of understanding—does not contradict its status as activity. The act of observation is simultaneously a sensorial exercise and also a type of semantic production that generates particular ways of seeing.

These two examples—the ethical[3] significance of interactive seeing and reciprocal visibility and the transition from aesthetic to contemplative observation—are sufficient to suggest that seeing is not adequately conceptualised when subjected to either realist or constructivist interpretation. The present investigation probes an alternative view of the problem by following the assumption that seeing is a practice and more specifically a performative practice entailing epistemic, ethical and aesthetic disclosure of the world. As a philosophical concept, *practice* has implications that permit seeing to be released from a subject-object schema. The term *world disclosure* designates a relation to self and to world involving understanding and interpretation. The claim is that visual perception is a performative practice with a world disclosing function similar to that of speech.

The term *world disclosure* refers not to a marginal aesthetic phenomenon within social practice. The example of visual communication between parents and children already indicates the existential significance of a world disclosing interpretation, including an ethical dimension. Just as world disclosure can be analysed, according to a Platonic and Kantian tripartite division, into a cognitive, an aesthetic and an ethical dimension, it can also be separated into linguistic and perceptually conditioned elements. Seeing can become world disclosure as the means by which we attain self-development and understanding of the world. This activity has a conventional dimension conditioning what we expect to see and are normatively expected (by society) to see. The individual dimension consists in creative displacements of common ways of perceiving something. In each of these cases, it is a question of a *mediating relation* in which opposites are yoked together into a more complex unity.

Just as Wittgenstein showed that spoken language consists of language games, forms of life and world disclosure, in a similar way the use of sight can be understood as eye witnessing, forms of life and world disclosure. Although the term *forms of life* is characteristically undefined in Wittgenstein, it can be understood as the practical character of seeing. Forms of life

[3]This book is founded on a broad notion of the ethical, encompassing those forms and situations of seeing involving the other and others, which make seeing and being seen morally and existentially significant instances of social visibility.

are the rule-giving context of possible experience, thought and action in a given society at a given time. They are the unquestioned given that must be accepted (Wittgenstein 1986, p. 200). Although collective conventions of seeing do not have the same status as fixed terms within a discursive language game, they too adhere to well-rehearsed interpretive schemata and are prefigured in the totality of valid norms and dominant mores. As such, they are additional constituents within the form of life of a cultural community.

It can be said that forms of life influence perception like coloured or magnifying glasses. In the same way, a general practice involving habitual ways of seeing and social visibility determines how something becomes visible and what it will be seen *as*.

A theoretical difficulty naturally arises here, since the lens itself cannot be taken in visually, at least not while it is being looked through. Forms of life are, like images of the world, the dispositional, implicit horizon of speech and perception that is never viewed in itself, although it is always part of the act of viewing. Nonetheless, in a theory of perception instructed by Wittgenstein's theory of language as usage, his insights can be applied to the use of the sense of sight; seeing is a practice embedded in a form of life, just as speech is. The context for this social sharing of a perceptual world is the entirety of historically and socially, publicly and institutionally recognised customs as well as dominant beliefs, interests and claims. The concept of practice makes it possible to suggest an alternative to both perceptual realism and constructivism.

The Aristotelian distinction between *poietic* and *practical* practice, between production of significance and activity that is an end in itself, can also be profitably applied to seeing in order to create a systematic order of the various ways of employing the term. The instrumental character of seeing as an act of knowledge is one such way. There is also a self-purposive or autotelic way of using sight, in which the person seeing and the thing seen are not necessarily opposed as subject and object. A distracted gaze is drawn to a visible entity capable of attracting attention, but the relation between the gazer and the entity would not be described as the deliberate or instrumental deployment of means. Seeing is an activity in two distinct respects: it has a pragmatic, purpose-oriented side and a practical, ethical side. Pragmatic seeing is involved in coping with practical demands of life. But seeing is not limited to this function. As a practice it is more, namely a way of disclosing the self, others and the visible world in the Kantian sense[4] of the practical exercise of freedom.

2 The Performativity of Speech and Sight

The main supposition underpinning this investigation is that seeing and speaking are analogous. Philosophy of language and speech act theory have shown speech to be more than mere information exchange and the simple statement of propositions. In the same way, a philosophical theory of perception illuminates the active and performative nature of perceptual world encountering.

Studies in philosophy of language have shown that language usage theory alone does not fully explain how language discloses reality. The compound of person, world and language are not static entities. The assumption that the three components exist independently prior to language, fails to account for the dynamics involved in any given performative act. The nominative speech acts involved in communication with others are mediated by symbols, while language is always already embedded in contexts of practical usage. If language were a static instrument, linguistic articulations could not generate their own objects or shape them creatively. The constitution of reality by consciousness would remain an obscure, if not entirely inexplicable process.

Perception is a similar case. Seeing is no more limited to constative seeing-that than speech is limited to propositional utterance. This comparison with speech helps explain the genuinely significant performative aspect of seeing. Just as speech is an act of realisation, so too can seeing be seen as an activity *in* which and *through* which the world is made to appear. As an activity effecting change in states of affairs, seeing has the character of a purposive tool; as an activity involving communication with others, it has the character of a mediated event.

[4] In the Critique of the Power of Judgment, Kant (2000) distinguishes the moral-practical from the technical-practical. The former means the unconditionally imperative, the latter the purposive deployment of means to ends (§88 and passim). A normative orientation on unconditional moral aims, as Kant demands it, can of course in no way be claimed for perceptual practice. However, the distinction is still useful for expressing the different types of rationality that are effective within practice: on the one hand, instrumental action oriented on the paradigm of efficient means to an end and on the other hand the moral demand of the end in itself.

An oversimplified notion of seeing as reality-replicating re-cognition and of the visible as objective presence, ignores the configuring and meaning-generating capacity of the act of seeing. Donald Davidson reminds us that we do not look *through* our eyes as through a telescope, we see *with* them.[5] In both activities, *how* speech and sight are enacted determines what is said and seen. Both speech and sight operate as performative practices, the nature of which is to *discover* a pre-existing reality while at the same time *constituting* that reality. Performance theory allows us to articulate this dual mechanism. In the performing of speech acts, reality and meaning are both produced and communicated. By the same token, perception encompasses a range of performative acts, such as communicative looking, with which concrete social effects are achieved (e.g., when issuing a warning or a demand), or self-purposive performances, in which process and result are indistinguishable from one another.

The practice of seeing is contingent upon context, which includes the act of seeing itself, as performed by the agent whose situation, mental and affective prerequisites individuate the perception. The way in which this performative agent performs speech and perceptual acts within the constraints of a given practice influences the sense and meaning of what is spoken and seen. Thus, the *how* of performance forms a part of its semantic articulation.

I draw on the term 'practice' insofar as it mediates between the subjective-constructive and objective-representational notions of seeing. The term 'performativity' is similarly used to mediate between notions of sight and insight. Views of the world involve choosing between different ways of understanding that world. Seeing is a highly selective and variable type of world disclosure because the act of seeing can be performed in so many different ways. An analogy between speech and sight is helpful, but there are marked differences between them. In visual perception, there is no medium comparable to the medium of speech and there is a larger gap between impression and expression, since the *how* of seeing remains an intrinsic procedure. Thus, the way relations to self and to world are mediated by perception should here be clarified, treating perception as a world-disclosing genre of its own, independent of mediation via language. The world is to the same extent given perspective by visual perception as it is mediated by spoken language.

[5] D. Davidson (1997, p. 18): "We don't look *through* our eyes, but *with* them."

The mutual interaction between language and perception also suggests the independence of the aisthetic. According to Humboldt, perception prefigures language use: "The whole way in which objects are perceived necessarily carries over into language use. Because words come into being precisely out of this perception, perception is not an imprint of the object in itself but rather the image the object generates in the soul." (Humboldt 1973, p. 53). Nor can perceptions ever be translated in full into utterances about perceptions.[6] Perceptions are indeed influenced and made possible by the words we have at our disposal.

Treating seeing in the same way in which speech act theory treats speech need not entail tethering it to a speech-like discursiveness. On the contrary, the aisthetic mode of relating to the world has its own proper, non-propositional sense, which needs to be worked out. Even in the case of communicative perception—for example, warning looks—the expression is anything but propositional. In cases such as Petrarch's perceptual relation to the world, his "numbness" at his aesthetic impression, and in everyday pragmatic seeing for the purpose of orientation, the non-linguistic quality is the essential feature.

In hermeneutics, the function of language in processes of interpretive world disclosure has been overestimated. What is *effectively* real in the real depends not on language alone but also on perceptions. Before something can be linguistically articulated, before the text of the world can be deconstructed, perceptions must be transposed into language. The "interpretive nature of humankind" (see Hogrebe 1992) begins with perceptions, not mainly with speech acts. An apprehension of being involves not primarily language; indeed, it is also image and picture.

Whether individual perceptions are understood as pre-reflective or whether emphasis is laid on their conceptual structure, they are not reducible to the speech paradigm. Whatever the interplay between speech and sight, they are neither deducible from nor can they be subsumed under one another. If visual perception must be understood as an organising principle of our relations to self and world, then it is its own genre of world disclosure. As such, the present book does not set out to pit language and perception against each other, nor to place one above the other. It is not about constructing a competitive model. The book engages rather in a complementary enterprise. Analogies can be established between language

[6] Martin Seel (2006) has provided some illuminating thoughts on this subject.

mediation and perceptual mediation that require closer examination. The fundamentally perspective-bound, plastic character of both these types of mediation needs to be investigated in terms of their aisthetic constitution.

3 The Double Sense of the Sense of Sight

The closeness of practical seeing to theoretical observation is demonstrated by the systematic connection of sight, insight, understanding, the formation of opinion, belief and knowledge. This proximity of the sense of sight to the mental processes of understanding, thinking and interpreting in practice consists in a dense intertwinement of seeing and ways of seeing as well as of sight and insight. When a child sees that they have angered their parents, they do not decode sensible evidence but rather see and understand at the same time. In the process, their act of understanding remains an act of seeing and not of hearing or imagining. In order to be able to explain such phenomena, we must assume that sight and insight are a unity. The likeness of the two terms cannot be treated metaphorically but must instead be taken literally.

The semantic field around seeing and its cognates exhibit a language-immanent density that is symptomatic of the complex problems surrounding vision. It reflects the difficulty of attempting to demarcate where seeing ends and something else begins. Our language use here indicates that intelligibility belongs to the sense of sight in a way that cannot be dismissed as simply metaphorical. The exacting observer *sees* through something—gains *insight*. The way someone is *regarded*, *respected*, depends on the *aspect* they offer to observers. The view one takes of things depends on how much one attains an *overview*, as well as what one *overlooks*. Someone casts a meaningful glance that says "*watch* out!" To disqualify all this as merely misplaced turns of speech would be to deny language any proper philosophical sense of its own and to fail to recognise the inevitability and indispensability of metaphor. In all the processes described, it is not possible to say definitively when seeing, looking and observing are sensible activities in the narrow sense and when an act of attention becomes thinking or interpretation. Seeing has a genuine double meaning. For this reason, talk of the lucidity of the sense of sight cannot be paraphrased in more literal terms; it is not an ornament for something that could just as easily be said more simply.

Just as puzzling as relations between the physical and mental, or between brain and mind, sensoriality and the sense of sight are caught up within a tension that cannot be resolved by building models of classification and hierarchical levels. To separate the visual process into a physiological and a mental activity is to ignore the factual unity of response and interpretation in that process. The double meaning must be captured not in terms of opposition or contrast but in terms of inter-permeable transitions. It thus requires parallel procedures. The method followed in this book therefore consists in thinking in analogies, similarities, comparisons and transferences—a "thinking that employs 'transitions' and keeps terminological borders porous" (Gabriel 1997, p. 370).

To this end, borrowings are made from very diverse theoretical contexts and terms need to be extrapolated heuristically. Relevant sources include the late Wittgenstein, with his linguistic considerations of seeing; and Merleau-Ponty, with his theory of perception. The figure of performativity from cultural studies will also be drawn from, as well as the anthropological term 'imagination' [*Einbildungskraft*]. This approach reflects the holistic character of perceptual practice. The notion of *seeing-as practice* contrasts with a model that distinguishes between taking account of something visually and adopting a mental attitude to it.

Analogical thinking provides the methodical key without which the polyvalence of the sense of sight is described too simplistically. We must proceed along multiple tracks in order to find out where seeing separates out into a state and an action. It is necessary to join together the various conscious acts involved in seeing while preserving their mutual differences in order to account for the way the visual and mental collaborate. In short, *seeing with other eyes* is both the object and the method of this book. The study abounds in transferences, comparisons and discoveries revealing similarities that enable a different way of *seeing* seeing. At the same time, disclosing the sense of sight by this method displays an analogue method of finding and inventing aspects and meanings.

4 THE ICONICITY OF VISUAL PERCEPTION

If performance theory can plausibly explain acts of perception as practically determined and, at the same time, determinative and constitutive, then a figurative, *presentative* element of expression is introduced into seeing. In other words, if perceptual world disclosure is an interpretive, picture- and mental image-making process—what I call 'iconicity'[7]—the question

[7]The terms 'image,' 'picture' and 'icon' each have varying definitions and connotations depending on context, which makes it difficult to choose one term over the other to suit all

becomes: what type of pictures are these, which both generate and inform perception at the same time? These pictures are not simply given as tangible objects but are rather instances of performance and its non-objective results; that is, perceived and imagined images that contribute to the idea we have of ourselves and the world.

An image is thus generally a special mode of the visual, since it is characterised by a self-reflecting instance of representation. As I will attempt to show, this applies not only to materially present pictures but also for immaterial images. Both are characterised by a particular relation between *what* is expressed in an image or representation and *how* it is expressed. The *how* is not a contingent, external form for the *what*, but rather determines what it specifically is. In this sense, images provide a sort of model for a characteristic of the performative practice of seeing: *how* someone sees something determines *what* will be visible. The perspective-bound structure of seeing *configures* the thing seen. In the case of non-objective perceptions and imaginings, this effect is of course a process entirely immanent to consciousness. As a rule, the pictorial, representational components of seeing are not themselves represented, but must instead be expressed in language or otherwise in order to become perceptible to others. Nevertheless, the act of seeing is in a certain sense comparable to linguistic expression; when someone sees *something-as-something* in a particular way, the modal *how* determines the semantic *what*. Ways of seeing relate to the object not separately, as a receptacle to its contents but rather seeing relates together with the object to constitute an inseparable compound of mutual conditions, such that altering the way of seeing alters the thing seen. The possibility of separating them theoretically must be presupposed, since the same object can be seen in many different ways. However, the two occur in practice as mutually interwoven. The theoretical account can only describe the practical whole by dividing individual elements, whereas in practice seeing and the seen condition each other. The *how* involves not only conclusions different from perception or simply capable of differentiation; it already involves an act of figuration within the performance of seeing.

Moreover, the pictoriality of perceptual practice is conditioned by the dimension of potentiality inherent in the visible. The visible is not simply identical with a present, objective world; it is not independent of the process by which it shows itself and is seen. It can go entirely unnoticed and appear

cases. For this reason, I will, at times, speak of 'iconicity' as an umbrella term to capture the pictoriality of images.

differently every time. A horizon of latent and possible visibility transcends what is actually seen at any one time. In what follows, the visible will thus be understood more as a disposition, an enabling ground for the ability to see than as the objective referent of the act of seeing.

This dispositional character means we need to integrate a notion of the invisible into our considerations. The invisible seems to inhere in the visible, not in the sense of an underlying 'essence,' but rather in that every act of vision is a particular combination of seeing and blindness. Expectations, additions and selective subtractions introduce a sensible absence into the event of seeing. When imaginings and interpretations come into play, seeing transcends its own bounds. The disclosure of the visible world must therefore take recourse to something invisible. Instead of invisibility, we could speak of *non-actualised perceptions* or of the *sensible non-present*. What is meant by this is that perception has a constant relation to other acts of consciousness, to memory and to inventive imagination.

The invisible distinguishes itself in a variety of ways; the imaginary and the imagined are not the same as the unseen sides of a die that seeing tacitly completes. The meaning attributed to something is a different kind of thing to an object too small or too distant to be detected by the human eye. The hidden is not simply something temporarily obstructed from view. In all these cases, however, the invisible is the horizon that needs to be there before the visible can appear to vision.

5 Ethics and Aesthetics

Perceptual practice has an aesthetic as well as an ethical dimension, in the sense that seeing and being seen are bound up with creative freedom and normative conditions. Our seeing takes place in the context of cultural customs and personal preferences. In seeing, the particular disposition of the individual, their tendency to see something one way instead of another way, transcend seeing itself and make it the constitution of a *viewpoint*.

Yet ways of seeing are at first immanent to consciousness and free from objectification. How perceivers represent something to themselves still has to be represented outwardly; for example, linguistically or deictically. This occurs paradigmatically in art, where a painter may bring a view of something into an image. In this way, an otherwise invisible performance becomes expressed in a sensibly perceptible way. What gets represented is *how* the artist saw *what* they saw. For this reason, one part of my reflections on seeing as performance uses studies of artworks to show how seeing, understood by the model of pictorial seeing, involves articulating representations. For their part, representations are ways of seeing that have become objects. Just as representations have their own unique style, our ways of perceiving the world could also be contingent on style. Like a personal style of handwriting, an individual *perceptual style* and a personal *visual ethos* could explain the space of free choice and the possibility of seeing differently, without which perception could not constitute world disclosure. Both reproductive and productive perception, the stereotypes and the variability of seeing, are conditioned by such representative styles of perception, from views of the world and styles of thinking.[8] The aspect of style is not a mere formal determinant; it is a moral factor that is manifested in the ethos and habitus of the seeing individual, whose biography and mentality structure the field of possible perception. This free range of visual possibility floating between creativity and convention presents the aporia that no general criteria can be laid down. However, in terms of the capacity of vision for world disclosure, the decisive characteristic is its pictorial nature.

The concept of performance alone is insufficient to explain the perceptual ability to produce images. We must refer to Kant, who posited the imagination, conceived as the 'faculty of images,' as an ingredient of perception (Kant 1998, p. 239). No theory of perception can do without such an image-making element. These two concepts—performance as a term from the theory of representation, and imagination as an anthropological faculty of representation (Kant 2000, §17, 23, 49, 62)—come from entirely different theoretical contexts, both of which serve to illuminate the dimension of seeing as a process by which perceptions come to constitute images of self and world. Such images are not to be construed as replicas of data otherwise present, but rather as indefinitely prolongable interactive processes enacted *between* mirroring and creation. In this in-between space, what can be seen and how it can be seen is decided by a variable and presumably never entirely determinable combination of perception and imagination, seeing and blindness, addition and subtraction, look and view.

[8] In a 1935 study, the physician and philosopher of science Ludwik Fleck (1981) coined the term 'style of thinking' ['Denkstil'] to describe sociological and historical influences on the development of scientific knowledge. For Fleck, a style of thinking is interestingly like a style of perception, "Seeing gestalt and seeing sense in terms of a style of thinking" are the forms of scientific observation that Fleck describes as stylised perception. The downside of collectively and individually influenced creativity in styles of thinking is thereby the danger of only seeing what we expect to see without contradiction and thus overlooking contradiction and otherness. I will return to this problem at various junctures.

I begin my investigation by eliciting the problems that have arisen from splitting seeing into receptivity on the one hand and intellectual spontaneity on the other. I further discuss possible alternative theoretical approaches (Chapter 2). The concept of practice provides a way out of the false dichotomy found in the history of metaphysics. In the web of relations joining persons in activity, perception (the actual) and the perceivable (the possible), are formed intersubjectively and interactively (Chapter 3). The concept of performance will explain seeing as an act not of arbitrary construction but of constitution that retains receptive and mediating features (Chapter 4). The relation between sight and insight poses a set of problems concerning the relation between the visible and the invisible (Chapter 5). The pictorial in acts of perception will be explained with the help of a concept of images and their genesis as processes influenced by the faculty of imagination, as discussed by Kant and Fichte (Chapter 6). In this way, the performance of seeing will be accounted for as an activity entailing realising and configuring effects that constitute self and world relations by means of perceptions and inner images. This leads to a discussion of the aesthetic freedom entailed by creative aspect-seeing and the ethical responsibilities involved in social visibility (Chapter 7).

The two final chapters provide concrete exemplifications[9] for testing the foregoing conceptual discussion. Sartre and Lévinas are cited in the case of an ethical distinction between seeing as instrumental identifying, and a seeing of personal acknowledgement. Sartre shows how one can look judgementally at the other and how the gaze can exercise power by fixing definitions. At the same time, Lévinas has made clear that non-dominance relations between the self and the other are enabled by the acknowledgement of an infinite and ungraspable difference (Chapter 8).

The aesthetic dimension will be demonstrated on the model of seeing art. In the experience of the artwork, we are confronted with visual material suited paradigmatically, in virtue both of its reflexivity and its character as act, to generate insights into the processes that weave together the visible and the invisible. The kind of seeing that both involves and represents art seems to me appropriate for considerations in the theory of perception, because of the way the artist sees and art works shape the visible world into a point of view that breaks with the routines of seeing as identifying. Art

[9] In the sense intended by Nelson Goodman (1976).

sets out systematically to see in different ways. This will be discussed with reference to Gary Hill (Chapter 9).

References

Austin, John Langshaw. 1962. *How to Do Things with Words: The William James Lectures Delivered at Harvard University in 1955*. Oxford: Clarendon Press.

Blumenberg, Hans. 1973. *Der Prozess der theoretischen Neugierde*. Frankfurt am Main: Suhrkamp.

Davidson, Donald. 1997. Seeing Through Language. In *Thought and Language*, ed. John Preston, 15–27. Cambridge: Cambridge University Press.

Fleck, Ludwik. 1981. *The Genesis and Development of a Scientific Fact*. Chicago: University of Chicago Press.

Gabriel, Gottfried. 1997. Logisches und analogisches Denken. In *Sprache und Denken*, ed. Alex Burri, 370–384. Berlin: De Gruyter.

Goodman, Nelson. 1976. *Languages of Art*. Indianapolis: Hackett Publishing Company.

Hogrebe, Wolfram. 1992. *Metaphysik und Mantik*. Frankfurt am Main: Suhrkamp.

Humboldt, Wilhelm von. 1973. *Schriften zur Sprache*. Stuttgart: Reclam.

Kant, Immanuel. 1998. *Critique of Pure Reason*. London and Cambridge: Cambridge University Press.

Kant, Immanuel. 2000. *Critique of the Power of Judgment*. Cambridge: Cambridge University Press.

Petrarca, Francesco. 1898. The Ascent of Mount Ventoux. In *The First Modern Scholar and Man of Letters*, 307–320. New York: Putnam.

Ritter, Joachim. 1989. Landschaft. In *Subjektivität*, 141–163. Frankfurt am Main: Suhrkamp.

Seel, Martin. 2006. Kenntnis und Erkenntnis. In *Die Artikulation der Welt*, ed. Georg W. Bertram et al., 209–230. Frankfurt am Main: Suhrkamp.

Thompson, Evan, and Noë, Alva (ed.). 2002. Introduction. *Vision and Mind: Selected Readings in the Philosophy of Perception*. Cambridge: MIT Press.

Wittgenstein, Ludwig. 1986. *Philosophical Investigations*. Oxford: Basil Blackwell.

CHAPTER 2

Why Seeing is a Problem

In the history of European philosophy, the question 'what is seeing?' tends to be interpreted in one of two ways. This polarisation structures the history of the concept from its very beginnings. The theories have oscillated dualistically since antiquity, and are biased towards one of the two poles of the event of seeing, either toward the *sensory* or toward the *sense-making* side of the process, either to the *receptivity* or to the *spontaneity* of the sense of sight. Moreover, sight is regarded as either advancing cognisance of the world or as the source of errors. These juxtapositions mirror a history of thought in which sight has been alternately ennobled as an instrument for gaining knowledge and disqualified as perfidious sensuality. Both notions have met with contradiction and objections, while themselves containing internal contradictions. The intellectualist devaluation of the sensory world goes hand in hand with the valorisation of an oculocentric logos.[1] Distrust of appearance is strangely contrasted with an almost blind trust in the indubitability of eyewitness accounts. Galileo's injunction to look through the telescope demands, on the one hand, that we trust the eyes and accompanying equipment, while on the other hand requiring us to doubt the immediate sensory impression. Because the insight that the earth is a rotating body

[1] Ralf Konersmann (1997, p. 23) has provided a lucid description of the contradictions inherent to both valorisations and devaluations of the faculty of vision: "Although Platonic-biblical thinking visualised the logos, the history of the ocular sense was not triumphal. The consistent intellectualist demand has been to deny acknowledgement to the appearance of the world."

E. Schuermann, *Seeing as Practice*, Performance Philosophy,
https://doi.org/10.1007/978-3-030-14507-1_2

does not follow from the ordinary sensory impression, but from knowledge and conclusions. Both, the mistrust of appearances and an unshakable belief in their authenticity, rest on the same epistemic model of sight, in which a subject *recognises*, *mirrors* and *pictures* an object, either by constructive activity or receptive passivity.

The emission theory of the ocular ray in optics as construed by Plato (see Simon 1992) first makes the claim for the productive character of vision before the Newtonian corpuscule theory or the wave theory of modern optics[2] demotes it to receptivity. However, whichever pole a theory favours, its antithesis quickly follows, such as when Aristotle's turn towards the empirical follows Plato's verdict against the illusory world of appearance—a verdict that Plato himself had already revised several times. The Protagorean maxim in the Theaetetus (152a-d) is that man is the measure of all things. Plato understands this to mean that being, as always already interpreted, cannot be mistaken by perception.[3] Similarly, picture-copy theories of seeing are countered by early forms of constructivism, such as that of Giambattista Vico. The reception theories, according to which seeing corresponds to the representation of a world as it exists independently of the process of seeing itself, are opposed to concepts of seeing as culturally coded (and therefore contingent on historical variations in the dominant patterns of interpretation) by which the productive processing of sensory impressions is integrated into seeing. In what follows, I offer a historical outline of the problems that have arisen from a conception of seeing within this dichotomy.

1 Oculocentrism and Its Critics

Several motifs reappear at almost every phase in the evolution of thought. From Descartes' Dioptric through Kant's anthropology to Jonas' claim of the "nobility of sight" (Jonas 1954), vision is regarded as the most aristocratic of the senses. The early proposition "nihil est in intellectus, quod non

[2] Gérard Simon describes optics since Descartes as "physics of light," The eyes cease to be the point of issue of an optic ray to become a camera obscura: "A camera obscura whose opening is the pupil, whose membrane is the iris, whose contractible camera lens is the crystal lens and whose screen on which the image appears is the retina" (ibid., p. 19).

[3] Gernot Böhme (2000, p. 203ff.) interprets Plato's theory of perception as a phenomenological. Indications of a correlation theory of perception, in which the entity seen and the entity seeing are mutually determined, can also be found in Plato (Theaetetus 159e-160a).

ante fuerit in sensu" recurs in various forms as the foundation of empiricist theories from antiquity to the nineteenth century. At the same time, the critical responses are just as emphatic in their underlining of the *unreliability* of the senses. While the critique extending from Plato to Hume is directed mainly against the propensity to deception in the sense of sight, in the twentieth century it is aimed at its real or presumed embroilment with power. Martin Jay's (1993) critique of ideology may overshoot the mark when he regards French philosophy as hostile to seeing. Merleau-Ponty at the latest belies this view. Nevertheless, his study makes it clear how central a role vision plays in the critique of rationalism in the twentieth century. The same goes, with some reservations, for David M. Levin's (1993) anthology. In Foucault's (1995) archaeology of historical modes of surveillance and the feminist critique (Irigaray 1985, 1987) of paternalistic conventions of seeing, the eye is suspected of being, above all, a virile instrument of domination. A frequent critique of ocular-centrism charges seeing with the violent appropriation of the other and others, as well as with a will to definition that both excludes and fixes. The gaze thus demonised bears an astounding historical similarity with its much older relative, the magic "evil eye" (Hauschild 1982). Under the label *phallogoculorcentrism*,[4] the phallus, the logos and the eye are regarded in equal measure as tools of the patriarchy. *Phallogoculorcentrism* ranges from the harassing to the excluding gaze, from objectification to repression, shutting out not only the feminine but all forms of otherness.[5] As pertinent as these diverse approaches are, they mainly testify to the fact that the will to power resides not in the eye as such, but in certain of its uses within specific contexts. Molestation and violence are not 'natural' tendencies of seeing but rather possible ways of using it to arrogate power within social constellations, suggesting above all that seeing must be regarded as a cultural practice. As Wittgenstein and the theorists of ordinary language have shown of speech, the meaning of seeing is contingent on its situation within the greater social framework. The implications of this will be worked out with the concept of practice.

[4]Luce Irigaray. Quoted in M. Jay (1992, p. 493).

[5]Very convincing in this respect is Kaja Silverman's (1997) treatment of the art of Cindy Sherman.

1.1 Epistemology and Hermeneutics

Epistemologists and practitioners of hermeneutics will give different answers to the question of what is seeing. The two approaches reconstruct the history of the concept in such fundamentally different ways as to seem to be dealing with different subjects. Each seems to have carved out their own terrain and then stopped paying attention to the other. This is evidenced in the two most recent German language anthologies on visual perception, which follow almost entirely disparate traditions. In the critical historical collection by R. Konersmann (1997), thinkers like Descartes, Locke, Kant and Husserl are omitted. In L. Wiesing's (2002) selection, there is no mention of Plato or Cusanus. Excepting Berkeley, Fiedler and Merleau-Ponty, both anthologies include entirely different thinkers. Anthologies must of course make a selection—they can only present excerpts and will contain gaps. A comparison of the two books nevertheless suggests that the epistemological and empiricist conception of seeing is simply incommensurable with a cultural studies/hermeneutic reconstruction of seeing, in which seeing is a socially and historically relative means of world disclosure.

The epistemological explanations generally concentrate on problems of the relation between seeing and judgement, perception and knowledge, beliefs and conclusions. A distinction is usually assumed between a foundational level of 'simple' or 'mere' seeing and higher-level judgement built on top of it. David Armstrong treats vision chiefly as the accumulation of information useful for acquiring knowledge: "Perception is nothing but the acquisition of true or false beliefs concerning the current state of the organism's body and environment" (Armstrong 1961).[6] Fred Dretske (1969) examines to what extent perception necessarily implies beliefs. For Searle (1983), having visual experience is fundamentally inseparable from the intentional belief that something or other is the case. Advocates of the distinction between perception and inference/judgement, mostly call on individual counter-examples but are unable to clarify in general terms the relation between perception and other mental acts, which are obviously bound up with perception and yet are distinct from it. The reason for this is that they restrict themselves mainly to conceptual analysis of the truth conditions of statements about seeing.

From the perspective of hermeneutics, such explanations are sterile, based on an artificial division of terms in relation to self and world that are

[6] A similar line of argumentation is found in D. C. Dennett (1991).

inseparable and work together. Heidegger writes that "any perception of useful things at hand always understands and interprets them" (Heidegger 1996, p. 140). Gadamer asserts that "pure seeing and pure hearing are dogmatic abstractions that artificially reduce phenomena. Perception always includes meaning" (Gadamer 2006, p. 92). Everything else is a formalism illegitimately laying claim to Kant. While the advocates of a theory of knowledge oriented toward scientific explanations accuse the hermeneutic version of confusing concepts, the notion of 'mere perception' is regarded by hermeneutics as reductionist.

These positions appear irreconcilable. But the difficulties lie not in arbitrary preferences or declarations of belief on the part of individual theoreticians. They are key to the question of the internal and external relations within which seeing occurs. The relation between sensibility and meaning, between seeing and thinking, is internal, whereas the relation between experience and world, inside and outside, subject and object, is external. The former is a problem of mind and nature, the latter of mind and culture.

1.2 The Idea of a Visual Deliverance

This leads to the most basic dualism in the history of the theory of vision. Like the oppositions between subject-object and sensibility-intelligibility, the naturalist and culturalist explanations are symptomatic of the traditional, hierarchical and binary interpretive framework. Most attempts to explain the sense of sight rely on dividing it into a lower layer of sensory receptivity and a more valorised layer of interpretive recognition.

Naturally, seeing can be described scientifically in terms of photons hitting nerve cells and triggering neuronal processes of a higher complexity, whereby the images from the retina are combined in the brain into a coloured image with spatial depth and connected to other faculties, i.e. memory and imagination.[7] However, social and semantic processes cannot be explained by descriptions of physiological processes in the brain and their subsequent cognitive computation.

[7] Irvin Rock (1985) has explained this in evolutionarily biological terms as the "intelligence of perception." See also Wolf Singer (2005, p. 148): "Our perceptions are not isomorphic pictures of some reality. They are instead the result of highly complex constructions and interpretation processes that rely heavily on stored knowledge." Picturesque renditions of the neurobiological wonders of vision are contained in David Hubel's (1988) compendium.

The act of speech is not usually described as mere transmission of sound waves later developing into an act of judgement by the posterior addition of meaning. Yet seeing is frequently held to consist essentially in retinal stimulus-response, whereas variations within the perception and attribution of meaning are regarded as not properly belonging to seeing itself.[8]

The historical dominance of this *myth of the given*, according to which the senses simply deliver material to thought, has complicated the problem. The antique and medieval division between *sensory eye* and *mind's eye*, the visio corporalis supplying the visio spiritualis with raw material to be elevated into intelligibility, rests on this paradigm and its naturalist logic. It has grounded sensualism at least since Condillac (1754), as well as sense data atomism[9] since Moore (1953). As the myth of the innocent eye, it has occupied art history since Ruskin.[10] It informs Jamesian (1950) sensationalism, Ayer's (1940) empiricism[11] and large chunks of Wolfgang Köhler's (1969) gestalt theory.

The assumption that there exist pure sense impressions depends on a theoretical distinction that does not occur in practice, placing seeing on the level of a culturally invariant, physiological, strictly ocular behaviour. Everything then that extends beyond sense impressions does not belong to the visible but to the mental—that is, to directed interpretation and knowledge. According to this view, we do not see people and houses,[12] but only colours and forms. This reduces the act of seeing to an optical reflex and the visible world to a type of neutral, physical *presence-at-hand* [Vorhandenheit] capable of being registered by complex machinery but incapable of being experienced by consciousness.

The notion of "mere perception" preceding the emergence of meaning, thought and knowledge, or "immaculate reception" [unbefleckte Empfängnis, i.e. Immaculate Conception] as denoted satirically by Nietzsche, is just as misguided as the notion that meaning is related to its

[8] Distinctions such as those made by Jerry Fodor (1990) between sense impressions and cognitively structured perceptions simply defer the problem.

[9] See the studies by M. Drechsler (1995) and Lambert Wiesing's (2002, p. 27ff.) commentary.

[10] The British art historian John Ruskin (1858) coined the expression "innocence of the eye" in connection with early modern painting. Ernst Gombrich (1960) has explained in detail, why there can be no such thing as an innocent eye. I will return to this in more detail.

[11] Austin (1962) critiques this from a linguistic viewpoint.

[12] This claim is made by R. Brandt (1999).

utterance as the content of a jug to the jug. Such a conception ignores the constructive part of speech acts. Yet treating not only linguistic expression but also visual perception as such an act of constructive articulation and form-making is generally regarded as mere rhetoric and metaphor, dressing up neuro-physiological processes in images. Standard philosophy of language does not divide speech into physiological and social-semantic layers as is done in the case of seeing.

There are, however, good reasons for the stubborn longevity of the myth of the given. Distinctions can be made between thinking and seeing, on the one hand, and seeing and the visible, on the other, that make the distinction between perception, thought and interpretation seem inevitable and imperative. This distinction is due in part to conventions of ordinary language use and theoretical description, and in part to everyday understanding. Both theory and common sense talk about seeing suggest the division. Since we have experiential evidence of external things that can be perceived in various ways, there seems to be a primary level of facts that are interpreted on a secondary level. More importantly though, interpretation talk presupposes the existence of something *for* interpretation that is logically and grammatically distinct from it. Whenever we have differing perceptions of the same object, we feel obliged to assume an activity of interpretation that can only be described by separating it analytically from perception itself. Whenever we speak of interpretation, we implicitly presuppose an object for interpretation in order to distinguish it conceptually from the contribution made by the act of interpreting. As such, the problems arising for any theory of perception partly stem from language use.

1.3 Aporias of Consciousness

The difficulties arise from the fact that seeing is an act of consciousness. Seeing becomes embroiled in all the usual problems of the theory of consciousness: the puzzling relation of mind to brain, the privacy of experience and questions of correspondence and accuracy in the relation between mind and world. Seeing is internally related to brain functions and processes of consciousness, as well as externally related to the visible, physical and social world. Because seeing is intentionally directed, it is closely bound up with mental states such as wishing, remembering and expecting and is extended to some object beyond consciousness. A series of questions—how objects for consciousness can emerge from physical and neural activity, how brain waves become perceptions of world, and how retinal images become views of the world—emerge as paradoxes of the internal relations of consciousness. *What* is given in experience, how much 'object' and 'subject,' how much world mind contains, is a question of the external relation of consciousness to the world.

The eye lies, so to speak, at the interstice between consciousness and world and is open to both sides. Locke's notion of the eye as window between the soul and the world is expressive of this peculiar medial location and the hybrid nature of vision. For him, the senses are "the windows by which light is let into this dark room" (Locke 1975, p. 115) of understanding. This imagery is misleading because it splits all acts of recognition into a subjective and an objective aspect. The two sides, once divorced, cannot be easily put back together. The divide between an intentional-representational and a material object of perception can never be closed again because there is no third standpoint from which to compare the two.

The notion of consciousness as a container into which recognition enters from without is so misguided that a concept of seeing based on it must end in aporia. With an ontology dividing subject and object, sense and sensibility into discrete substances, there is only the choice between a theory of perception as radically interpretive and one of simple representationalism. It is irrelevant whether representations are regarded as standing for material things or simply as mental entities. The generative and interpretive aspects of seeing are unexplainable on the presupposition that understanding is, as Locke states, "not much unlike a closet wholly shut from light, with only some little opening left, to let in external visible resemblances, or ideas of things without" (Locke 1975, p. 115). This means we perceive whatever is 'given' to vision, with no freedom to see differently. Inversely, the presupposition of a 'purely subjective seeing' leads to an equally implausible, unsharable and incommunicable private world.

1.4 Revenants from the History of Metaphysics

The old conflict in metaphysics between empiricism and rationalism, between realism and scepticism is repeated in the twentieth century in the conflict between phenomenology and constructivism. The same questions emerge: how much world does the mind contain; how does sensibility become sense and significance; and what is given in experience?

The associated questions are among the most controversial in the history of philosophy: is the sense of sight directed towards 'things as they are' (as some phenomenologists assume), or to mental representations (which entails the problem of hypostasis); to a 'natural reality' (which the sense data theorists must buy into despite all efforts at avoidance); or to semiotic image and text-like processes? On the one hand, the sensualist defence of cognisance supported by experience seems reductionist. On the other hand, theories according highest priority to the element of construction in seeing risk depriving it of the capacity to contain world.

Strangely, dogmatism and scepticism are affiliated forms of empiricism. Into the twentieth century, in the positivism of Neurath and Carnap, as well as in parts of Husserl's phenomenology, the claim to experience as the incontestable foundation of knowledge failed to avoid the twin extremes of dogmatic realism and sceptical doubting of subjectivity. On the one hand, sense experience is held to be a reliable foundation, containing 'reality' or 'things as they are.' On the other hand, the admission of differences between perception and its objects inevitably leads to a problem of mediation.

Talk of the given in both experience and phenomena is the same type of talk, as Susanne Langer has surmised: "when we speak of the 'given,' of 'sense data,' 'the phenomenon' or 'other selves,' we take for granted the immediacy of the external world. Our fundamental questions are framed in these terms: What is actually given to the mind? What guarantees the truth of sense-data? What lies behind the observable order of phenomena? What is the relation of the mind to the brain? How can we know other selves? [...] Their answers have been elaborated into whole systems of thought: empiricism, idealism, realism, phenomenology, Existenz-Philosophie, and logical positivism" (Langer 1979, p. 10).

1.5 The Necessity of Mediation

To what extent Kant's distinction between concepts and sense intuitions is responsible for the myth of the given is a pertinent question, since it forces us to reflect on the problems above. In one sense, the main function of Kant's theory of the faculties of cognition is to explain the interaction and mutual conditioning of sensibility and understanding. At the same time, what is supposed to be demonstrated as inseparable is attributed to distinct faculties; whence the need for the schematism chapter in the *Critique of Pure Reason* and finally Kant's further elaboration of the faculty of judgement in order to explain the connection between thought and perception. A complex interplay of the imagination and judgement as mediating faculties is needed to reconcile the faculties of knowledge, which are otherwise in danger of drifting apart. Konrad Fiedler (1991) was not entirely on the wrong track when he critically set apart his Expression Theory of Sensibility from the notion of sensibility as the deliverer for thought, which he attributes to Kant. Fiedler's reproach is aimed at the notion that sensibility is merely the unstructured raw material for conceptually structured knowledge. S. Majetschak has explained Fiedler's objections in terms of a hierarchy of priorities in Kant's thinking. "The categories regard the intuition of an object only in so far as thought requires it for judgement. They do not develop the intuition as intuition, but rather represent the given as 'judgement serving'" (Majetschak 1989, p. 279).

Kant's position shows the inevitability of the aporias, demonstrating that the bipolarity of the two faculties must be invoked even in the attempt to demonstrate their unity. Although well aware that intuition without concepts is blind and concepts without intuition are empty, Kant is unable to avoid assuming the existence of a "pure intuition." His difficulty is a symptom of the hiatus between a practical whole and its theoretical dissection. In order to bridge this gap, it is necessary to employ mediating concepts of process.

1.6 Problems of Reference

The question of the *fundamentum in re* for seeing was traditionally addressed by causal theories involving either physical or neural causality. The model of a monocular observer,[13] modelled on the camera obscura and usually attributed to Descartes,[14] can be seen as an example of a causal theory. The same can be claimed for various versions of mental representationalism. Both the rationalist and empiricist models hold that we see images of things, not the things themselves—except that in the former case, the images are caused by mental entities and in the latter case by external objects. The rationalists hold that consciousness reacts to its own states, while the empiricists assert that it reacts to the corresponding objects. According to one of the various concepts of representation used by Locke, mental representations are ideas *of* consciousness or *in* consciousness and are apprehended by perception: "Consciousness is the perception of what

[13] Jonathan Crary (1988) made an interesting comment on this, comparing the Cartesian observer to the observer from Goethe's colour theory.

[14] Ralf Konersmann (1995) has cast doubt on this attribution.

passes in a man's own mind" (Locke 1975, p. 115). Ideas are effects of things on consciousness. A fata morgana is sense data without a material referent, and knowledge of this fact cannot be taken from perception itself (see Ayer 1940). Berkeley's (1948) phenomenalism is based on this assumption that visual perception is entirely self-referential.

Causal theories, as advocated in the twentieth century by Strawson (1979)[15] and Grice (1957), among others, assume that visual impressions are caused by material objects in the world. Although this notion is intuitively convincing, it buys into the difficulty of explaining knowledge as adequation. If the object of perception is separable from perception itself, there must exist an ontological referent compared to which the act of consciousness can be either more or less adequate.

The issue at stake in these questions of reference is no less than the adequacy or correspondence of thought, speech and perception to "what there is" (Quine 1953a). These problems still drive analytic philosophy today. From Quine's (1953b) pragmatic critique of the dogma of immediate experience to Davidson's interpretationism, from Sellars to McDowell, the task has been to understand the relation of mind to world and the validity of statements about this relation. Sellars (1956) designated the false approach to this problem as the myth of the given, casting doubt on the validity of sense data theories of perception.[16] McDowell (1994) took this further by describing how experiences already have conceptual content. This linguistic turn in empiricism consigns the mediated character of relations to self and world to the conceptual. From this viewpoint, "we are placing it in the logical space of reasons, of justifying and being able to justify what one says," writes McDowell (1994, p. xiv) quoting Sellars.

Richard Rorty claims to avoid the problem by getting rid of the paradigm of correspondence: "The choice is between dropping the notions of 'answering' and 'representing [...] and keeping them" (Rorty 1998, p. 135). To keep them is to stabilize authoritarian structures, as (according to Rorty) does Brandom; "I see Brandom's persistence in using the terms 'getting right,' 'really is,' and 'making true' as tools that will fall into authoritarian hands and be used for reactionary purposes" (ibid.). Finally, however, Rorty cannot make a convincing case for how we should do away with such expressions altogether. Correspondence seems to be, as W. Welsch (2000,

[15]Strawson's critique of the correspondence theory of truth seems to refer primarily to talk about perception, not to perception itself.

[16]Sellars attack is directed less at the conception of sense data than the validity of arguments based on sense data.

p. 21) writes, "a tumbler that always bounces back [...], and so can't be gotten rid of that easily."

This is, however, not the place to reconstruct the debate in all its complexity. Of chief importance for the faculty of vision is the insight that examining seeing in the light of epistemological premises lands you in a nest of difficulties with its own rich tradition.

It will be discussed later whether or not the problem is merely deferred by Merleau-Ponty's (1962, p. 46ff.) suggestion of connecting seeing and the entity seen by motivation rather than by causality, according to which a phenomenon is capable of arousing attention. The same doubts apply to interpretation theories, such as Goodman's, that perception consists in processes of sign mediation. I will attempt to show that it is helpful, when operating within a notion of seeing as practice, to assume the existence of *styles of perception* informing what is seen and how. Just as a figurative style is not primarily determined by the object but rather by the artistic expression of the form of figuration, perception would thus not be determined by the perceived but, at most, occasioned by it. The concept of style can only be explained plausibly within a conception of seeing that borrows from theories of representational expression.

However, even with the aid of such notions, the antipodes of metaphysics cannot be escaped entirely, if for no other reason than the fact that grammar obliges us to think in terms of subject and object. If a relation is assumed between consciousness and world as between two distinct substances, there is only an either-or choice. Either the person seeing constitutes what they see, in which case all sceptical objections hold, or they claim a given and are exposed to the charge of pre-critical essentialism. This is a clear indication as to which aporias the question of seeing leads when regarded as a fundamental concept in epistemology and considered under the premises of a representationalist paradigm. The epistemic ideal of neutral perception necessarily leads in the wrong direction. It is just as misleading as the presupposition that the visible is a given that already exists independently and then appears or is seen as something—that is, as something other than what it is. The dichotomies *content and form*, *perception and perceived* split a practical, mediated process into a false dichotomy, replacing a holistic set of interrelations with a relation of containment of the one by the other. The concept of practice promises a frame of reference escaping this polarisation. The use of language entails certain antinomies, conflicting principles, *between* which perception is performed. The practical unity of the visual and the mental is indeed based on their conceptual distinguishability.

1.7 Knowing, Believing, Concluding

This fact can easily be demonstrated using the example of Nelson Goodman's interpretationism. The attempt to show the connectedness of terms whose disparity needs to be presupposed almost inevitably leads to performative self-contradiction. When Goodman writes that the eye is dependent on "intimations" from the other senses, the "heart" and the brain, he seems at first to assume a reduction of seeing similar to that of sense datum theories. He then proceeds to draw the entirely different conclusion that since seeing is always involved in social and individual contexts it is not culturally invariant and natural, but rather a symbolically mediated and mediating activity. He must presuppose the very "optical perception," which he at the same time refutes. "The eye comes always ancient to its work, obsessed by its own past and by old and new insinuations of the ear, nose, tongue, fingers, heart, and brain. It functions not as a self-contained instrument, but as a dutiful member of a complex and capricious organism. Not only how but what it sees is regulated by need and prejudice. It selects, rejects, organizes, discriminates, associates, classifies, analyses, constructs" (Goodman 1976, pp. 7–8).

There is clearly a contradiction between the unity and disparity, the connectedness and separateness between seeing and other conscious behaviours. Even when Goodman (1978, p. 71) writes that it would not have been possible to see "the football trainer" without knowing that the man on the far right is the trainer, he seems to paradoxically posit something within seeing that exceeds seeing. Who or what the trainer is is indeed not a matter of visibility. Social roles and functions are not themselves visible. Nevertheless, one can see that the person who appears to be the trainer has something to say to the players who in turn follow his directions. In the context of intersubjective and/or social practice, something becomes visible against the background of something invisible, like a figure against a field. Seeing unfolds between the visible and the invisible as a mediating movement. The relation between seeing and knowledge consists not in a one-sided act of delivery but rather a relation of mutual conditioning, in which knowledge is arrived at via seeing and, at the same time, we are only able to see what we know.

According to the currently accepted version, knowledge arises from observation, memory and induction. Empirical knowledge is judged certain when the sense impressions of various modes of perceptions are mutually consistent and recur reliably. When I see apples hanging on a tree and conclude that I am standing in front of an apple tree, I then see the 'apple tree' as such for the first time as a result of drawing the conclusion. Without the corresponding botanical knowledge, I would not have read from the tree that type of tree it is but would nevertheless have had the perception of a tree. The belief that I am seeing a tree is due not just to what is seen but also the inference *from* seeing the apple. If I have *learnt* from this what an apple tree looks like, the next time I encounter an example of this genus I can legitimately be said to be seeing an apple tree rather than just having a blind—that is, meaningless—sensory intuition bereft of real knowledge.

In Searle's (1983) example, when Jones sees a yellow station wagon, but does not know that it is a yellow station wagon, the distinction between seeing and knowing is based on a third standpoint that compares the first two. As long as this *tertium comparationis* is possible, perception can be distinguished from other mental activities with relative ease without having to assume a hierarchical relation between a meaningless sensory apparatus and operations of thought generating meaning. It is fundamentally reductive to assume that perception is devoid of judgement. Nevertheless, impressions can occasionally be distinguished from inferences. In such cases, it can make sense to disconnect the mental from the visual. This can be done, however, without squeezing the visual into a sensualist atomism. For example, a true impression can lead to false conclusions. Inversely, factually correct conclusions from seeing can depend on incidental circumstances.[17] Phenomena like the apparently broken rudder in water or the Müller-Lyer illusion are instances of perceptions that can subsist independently of the perceiver's contrary knowledge.[18]

Yet many of these cases rest on elliptical turns of speech. We do not, strictly speaking, *see* 'clouds driven onward by the wind' but just clouds in motion. Is it possible to actually *see* a 'bank robbery' or do we just see masked, menacing-looking figures in a bank?

A logically more complicated question is: what do we see when we see that someone we are waiting for at the station is not there? In this context, not-seeing-something amounts to seeing-something.

[17] See W. Künne's (1995) sophistic example of a bald man wearing the mask of a bald man in order to conceal a scar. The judgement is correct that the man is bald, although the sense impression involves an illusion.

[18] Ralph Schumacher's (2004) Reconstruction of Berkeley convincingly shows that Berkeley's theory of perception is capable of explaining why some perceptions can display such independence from beliefs, despite the fact that perception is fundamentally subject to the influence of experience and habits.

Whether the fact that someone sees something justifies the assumption that they will arrive at an associated belief can be determined only in individual cases and never with final certainty.[19]

1.8 *Seeing Something, Seeing That, Seeing How*

Seeing should certainly be understood as accessing the world by means of recognition leading to conclusions about the way visible things are and developing opinions that something or other is the case. It is wrong, however, to confine the range of what can count as seeing and to let drop all the significant differences between the other forms of seeing. Seeing is presumably always a synthetic, practical behaviour of the eyes involving elements of blindness, but it is certainly not a propositional act of identifying that such and such is the case. Not even all instances of seeing-that can be grasped as seeing in the constative, epistemic sense, since what is the case is a question of the way you look at it. The example of the child that sees *that its parents are angry* shows that not all seeing-that can be regarded as an act of unproblematic recognition and that more complex cases should not be regarded as seeing only in a metaphorical sense. Seeing *that* my child is growing up is not perceivable in the same way as seeing *that* it is wearing blue trousers. The presence of something blue in the sense of a phenomenon of a specific wavelength can be measured by an appropriate device, but the child's growing up is not determinable by technical means. Even if recognising the colour were taken as a largely unproblematic case of constative seeing, this would still not explain all perception. In the course of his considerations, Austin himself casts doubt on his own distinction between performative and constative speech acts[20] according to which there can exist purely constative speech or, for that matter, sight.

Seeing may contribute decisively to knowledge in certain cases, even in a great many. Yet these are special cases of aesthetic and communicative seeing. It is problematic to equate cognitive seeing with intentionality and propositionality. Searle is probably the most prominent advocate of this

[19] Dretske (1969, p. 20) contests that the utterance "that D looks some way to S" also means "for some character C, it looks to S as though (as if) D (or something) were C," which would imply the existence of a form of non-epistemic seeing. His plea for a distinction between perception, beliefs, opinions etc. is however in large part founded on the contrary claim: "D can look some way to S without it looking to S as though it were C (for any C)."

[20] S. Krämer (2003) has commented on this insightfully, also in (Krämer 2001).

equivalence, placing seeing-that, seeing-something and intentionality in the same box: "From the point of view of Intentionality, all seeing is seeing that: whenever it is true to say that x sees y it must be true that x sees that such and such is the case. [...] The fact that visual experiences have propositional Intentional contents is an immediate (and trivial) consequence of the fact that they have conditions of satisfaction, for conditions of satisfaction are always that such and such is the case" (Searle 1983, p. 40ff.).

Seeing p is equivalent to seeing-that-p. When I see a black piano I also see *that* the piano is black. I then come to the conclusion and the belief that the piano is black. This state of belief can be translated into a proposition of the type a = b, is thus subject to truth criteria and thereby admitted to the procedures for validating correctly formed judgements.[21] Propositional seeing therefore, like predicative speech, performs specific attributions of identity. This propositional seeing is regarded, implicitly or explicitly, both in ordinary language and in theoretical discourse, as the most general and fundamental form of visual perception.

The great majority of cases can indeed be well described within this framework. Cognisant seeing-that is presumably the most common case of seeing in everyday experience. But this tells us absolutely nothing about the qualitative *how* of seeing. Those states of mental experience referred to in the philosophical debates as qualia are indeed conditioned by perception, or rather by performance,[22] but they are not propositional.[23] Seeing how something looks cannot in all cases be transposed into utterances capable of being subjected to truth criteria and is therefore neither intentional nor propositional.[24] Seeing-how is a case of non-propositional and non-intentional seeing that could be referred to as epistemic in individual cases but does not function as a type of utterance.

There is a further difference here, the importance of which is often underestimated. *Seeing-something* need not entail *seeing something-as-something* or *seeing something-in-something*. Seeing the station wagon does

[21]This aspect of epistemic seeing is also heavily emphasised by R. Chisholm (1957).

[22]In that they depend on the performance of an act of seeing. Cf. III.1.a)-c).

[23]On the concept of non-propositional cognisance and thought, see G. Gabriel (1997) and C. Schildknecht (1999).

[24]Christiane Schildknecht (2003) has argued that because there exist non-conceptual sense impressions, we should make a distinction between content of perception and content of conviction, qualifying the way an object looks as something that is irreducible to propositional content.

not mean seeing it *as* a station wagon and seeing a cloud is not the same as recognising the contour of a figure in the cloud.[25] In other words, the *intentionality* of seeing is entirely distinct from its propositionality.

1.9 Conclusions

It should have become clear by now that separating seeing into a basic form of registering receptivity on the one hand and intelligent spontaneity on the other artificially portions out the problem and loses sight of its wholeness. Seeing is so tightly interwoven with mental activities and with a series of evaluative behaviours such as imagining, believing, fearing and judging as to be more appropriately grasped as a practical form of world disclosure than as a vehicle of acquiring knowledge.

The solutions worked at by the authors treated above deserve closer examination. Any cursory consideration of many of these historical positions necessarily remains superficial. However, such an overview of basic features in the history of the concept is aimed not at the individual authors but seeks instead to reconstruct the problem from a particular systematic standpoint. The intention is to show that basic empiricist, epistemic and representationalist concepts are not complex enough to explain seeing. The terminology of representation leads to the false alternative between pre-critical essentialism and relativist interpretationalism. A different approach is needed in order to understand how we function within the world by means of seeing.

In the practice of seeing, there is a continuous cooperation of elements that theoretical description artificially divides up. The act of seeing itself can only be separated forcibly into conceptual and perceptual components. A different terminology is needed to mediate the dualism. Understood as performative practice, seeing is a situated activity involving both making determinations and being determined. As a conscious act it is a two-sided activity involving consciousness and world. The opposition between inner and outer cannot be abandoned entirely because it will always be necessary to assume an internal relation of consciousness in seeing as well as an external relation to world, despite the difficulties this distinction entails.

[25] M. Seel (2004) has pointed out that seeing-something-in-something is not even the same as representative or iconic seeing. Seeing faces in clouds or wall marks does not mean they have been represented there.

Instead of grasping the two-sidedness of perception as a disjunctive either-or relation of rival priorities, it would be more advisable to choose the more reserved *neither-nor*. Pure constructivism is just as unfounded as pure sensibility. Seeing is not a neutral channel for imbibing information, nor is the visible world a blank screen for all sorts of projections. Despite the importance of selection and individuality in perception and the contributions of the imagination, affects and associations, we do not live in private worlds that we cannot share with others.

As we have seen, there are systematic reasons for assuming that seeing implies opposite poles of reception and invention, taking-in and making, mirroring and constructing, and that these poles require mediation. The terms 'performativity' and 'practice' will need to be tested for their ability to explain the way seeing mediates between the visible and the invisible, the real and the possible. The most important part of this is to avoid thinking of these oppositions as object-like entities within a substance-ontology, and instead to consider them as the moving parts of a dynamic process constituting a practice—a practice within a form of life and where opposites are mediated.

Consequently, this book will be unable to avoid assuming certain dualisms as the extreme poles of an activity that in fact always takes place in the interstices. However, these poles will be regarded as practical connections and not as the hypostatic sides of a puzzling correlation. New perspectives could be opened by considering seeing in the light of H. Plessner's notion of "mediated immediacy"—this is, as a type of relation that is neither purely immediate nor entirely mediated, playing out in an in-between space cohabited by over-determination and indeterminacy, the gaze and the point of view, impression and expression.

2 Other Approaches

There are various theoretical points of departure for approaching these considerations. In what follows, Cassirer's theory of symbolic forms will be shown to be just as stimulating as interpretation theory, and both semiotic and narrative theories will also be drawn upon before finally, albeit with a different emphasis, considering approaches from the realm of visual cultural studies.

2.1 Symbol Theory

Cassirer's theory of symbolic forms is basically a theory of cultural world disclosure. My investigation is provided with a point of contact by the notion "that the 'understanding' of the world is no mere receiving, no repetition of a given structure of reality, but comprises a free activity of the spirit" (Cassirer 1957, p. 13),[26] due as much to the imagination as to sense perception. Another useful idea is his description of self and world relating as expressions of active conscious processes[27] by which the individual becomes an animal symbolicum, which "has a world of its own because it has an experience of its own" (Cassirer 1962, p. 23).[28]

Cassirer develops a theory of culture as a form of activity[29] entailing, in a practical sense, a relatedness both to one's self and to the world. He remains constantly aware of the affective and imaginative tincture of this type of relation without discrediting it as irrationalism. "Man does not live in a world of hard facts, or according to his immediate needs and desires. He lives rather in the midst of imaginary emotions, in hopes and fears, in illusions and disillusions, in his fantasies and dreams" (Cassirer 1962, p. 25). Reality is never immediately given, but always mediated, interpreted, structured. The universe of symbolic forms such as language, art, religion, philosophy and science is a practical manifestation of understandings of the world that have assumed tangible shape in symbols. The place of perception in this universe is as the "view" from a sense whose nature is to be sensually embodied. The visible is "never outside a specific type of 'vision' and cannot be thought apart from it. As sensual experience it is always already the bearer of sense" (Cassirer 1957, p. 200). In the same vein, Susanne Langer

[26] For an updated version, see E. W. Orth (1992).

[27] On Cassirer's conception of consciousness and the parallels to Husserl's concept of intentionality, see M. Plümacher (2004).

[28] Cassirer occasionally loses sight of his own insight when he disconnects this self-sufficient world of perception from the "world of sense impressions" in which we touch merely the "surface of reality" (ibid., p. 169).

[29] See B. Recki (2004, p. 26). Recki reconstructs Cassirer's concept of culture as "the medium of our poietic-practical self interpretation." However, the performativity of this self and world interpretation is receiving increasingly less attention. The emphasis is instead placed on its normative connections to the values and rules of a language community.

(1979) refers to seeing as an act of formulation. The fullness [*Prägnanz*] of perception gives form to the symbolic fullness of a sign.[30]

With all due respect to this comprehensive and profound work, the reader cannot dispel certain discontents and suspicions. Despite protestations to the contrary, Cassirer's epistemological point of departure and his chief distinctions—namely mental content/sensible form; sensible, perceptual experience/insensible, non-perceptible sense; form/matter—are dangerously close to becoming static substances. The analytical necessity of such distinctions hinders the appropriate treatment of their interpenetration. It is frequently emphasised that no content can be thought without form and vice versa, but in Cassirer's work their interrelation reads unavoidably as a relation of containment. This is partly due to the theoretical necessity of exhibiting them separately while desisting from systematically building on this separability. The term 'performativity' seems to me capable of navigating around such cliffs. Cassirer was no early performativity theorist. The paradox of a foundational mediation or a responsive constitution could only be reformulated within his theory against the resistance of the representations and objectifications entailed by cultural signification.

2.2 *Interpretation Theories*

In the theory of seeing as a world-disclosing practice, perception theory intersects with hermeneutics, semiotics and interpretation theory (see Abel 1993; Simon and Stegmaier 1994). Even a constructivist theory of knowledge works with similar axioms. Popper, for example, writes that facts show up only in the light of theory. Facts relate to their perception not as being to appearance. Instead, different views of the facts disclose those facts in such a way as to give them a specific shape. These processes could thus be explained within the framework of interpretationism. The concept of world disclosure needed for a theory of seeing is close to the concept of interpretation. World disclosure is one of a variety of cognitive ways of relating to the world. When we see the world, we are also already interpreting it. Every interpretation extends, as E. Angehrn explains, from "the

[30]Oswald Schwemmer's (1997) work is helpful here in explaining the ethico-aesthetical connection between form-giving and form-becoming. The concept of an interaction between a form formans and a form formata in Cassirer's posthumous writings could supply an appropriate basis for a reformulation of his ideas in terms of performance theory.

indirect understanding to subjective determination and object constitution" (Angehrn 2003, p. 146). It follows from this that the interpretation itself, whether linguistic or aisthetic, already displays that double meaning of responsiveness and which is constitutive of seeing. The interpretation can be "constitutive or posterior, universal or particular, constructive or reproductive-receptive" (ibid.). As the development of a way of seeing, vision is an interpretive act.

It is preferable nevertheless to explain these complications in terms of world disclosure because both the hermeneutic and deconstructionist concepts of interpretation are dedicated to the treatment of texts. The iconicity of the aisthetic is a quality in its own right, distinct from the textual form of language. Its visuality should therefore not be neglected. Perception can only be world disclosure when it is tied up with other mental operations like analysis, interpretation, understanding, expectation, imagination and conviction.

Different authors have employed various modifications of the term. For Heidegger, world disclosure is the basis of all relations to self and world. For Habermas, it is the aesthetic margin of a social practice (see Kompridis 1993). Rorty (1989) has described world disclosure as a movement between invention and discovery.

Against Heidegger and Habermas, Martin Seel (2002, p. 45) has jettisoned the concept of "world disclosure as a term opposed to truth and validity," developing it instead as a "process of erosion and revision" that "shakes the fixed notions of a certain matter together with their supporting points of view and standards" (ibid., p. 54). This transformative quality of encountering the world was also emphasised by Dewey. With reference to Dewey, I want to use the concept to mean a creative form of interaction with the world, which opens parts of that world by producing new ways of looking or by transforming old ones. This usage is distinct from the constructivism implied by Goodman's concept of worldmaking.

Most theories understand world disclosure on the basis of a continually situated involvement, which is pre-structured holistically, pre-reflexively and grammatically. We find ourselves in a world we already partly understand. Its horizons of meaning are already always disclosed. This is why no final world disclosure is possible, whereas new forms of seeing, hearing and interpreting always remain possible, not least by means of art.

In what follows, the word *disclosure* will be used to emphasise the character of a process. The disclosed world needs to be generated in performance and with a particular *manner* of disclosure. The world cannot be regarded as already there and accessible in a substance-like, essentialist sense without regressing to objectivism. Something or other must already actually be there for it to be disclosed, but this something is as indeterminate and inaccessible as the Kantian thing-in-itself.

Seeing can become world disclosure when it is the means by which a view of the world is constituted. The conventional dimensions of this activity are manifest in our expectations and customs of seeing, the individual dimensions in creative divergences from expectations and customs.

2.3 *Narrative Theories*

While recourse to speech act theory is fundamental to the present book, a further point of comparison may provide insights: the perceptual disclosure of the world could possess a similarly *iconic* constitution to the narrative, linguistic mediation of world. In other words, speech could be to narrative what seeing is to the image.

Since Dilthey and Heidegger, philosophy has been attentive to the processes by which the self and external reality are constituted by means of narrative. A whole range of narrative theories (e.g., A. MacIntyre 2007; Rorty 1989; Taylor 1985) have been drawn upon to render comprehensible the indissoluble relations of practice and speech to explanation and understanding, interpretation, story-telling and representation. According to Hannah Arendt (1959, p. 164.), "sharable stories are the genuine 'products' of action and speech." Heterogeneous events, actions and experiences are joined to make a more or less coherent whole—that is, a story, with a *before* and an *after*, by means of the plasticity of narration. As Ricoeur (1984, 1985, 1988) has shown, narrative gives shape to time itself.[31] Lived time becomes life story, providing in some circumstances a justificatory account of that life.[32] With their language and their perceptions, humans

[31] Ricoeur seems to me to somewhat uncritically overestimate the role of narration in developing order and founding unity. His classical leading figure is Odysseus on the way to himself and finally arriving. The errors and losses on this journey of self-discovery are generally blocked out.

[32] The advantages and disadvantages of this transformation for personal relations to the self are explored by Dieter Thomä (1998). Thomä approaches the subject from the question: What is right living? Narrative is a more appropriate way to develop an adequate image of one's own life than the traditional projects of self-recognition. Although narrative can never answer the leading question, it can help "to experience, how I am and to construct what is important to me about me" (ibid., p. 15).

are self-interpreting creatures. Narrative is a *form of representation* for practice. It has not only aesthetic meaning but also a justificatory, ethical function. As Charles Taylor has shown, in narratives of actions, the actors' reasons and motives can be made explicit in different ways, entailing different interpretative descriptions.[33]

Narrative theory naturally lays the greatest emphasis on the linguistic nature of relations to self and world. I would like to direct our attention to the iconicity of these relations, that relies not only on linguistic acts of articulation but is the result of a multitude of aisthetic acts. The interpretive character of narrative images of self and world, their variability and plasticity can be articulated in speech in order for it to be communicated between subjects, but is unthinkable outside of a plurality of different types of aisthetic occurrences. The procedures of fiction by which individuals bestow narrative form on themselves and their lives are pre-figured in perceptual phenomena. Narratives are based on perceptions; perceptions of ourselves, our world and the others involved in our life stories. In turn, perceptions involve imagination. Expectations and previous experiences permeate perceptions and condition what can enter into view and become an object of attention. Acts of perception and imagination sweep on before the moment of narration where experience hardens into story-telling. They constitute iconic preconditions for the narrative and aesthetic constitution of identity. The aesthetic reveals herein its aisthetic origins. The material perception is not simply registered but formed into a *perceptual image*, dependent not only on what is visible but also on invisible contextual factors, circumstantial conditions as given by the times, the environment and other background phenomena. The iconic character of perceptions is conditioned by these background factors. The moments of articulation in relation to self and world derive from image and sound as well as from text and word and their affective efficacy may therefore derive primarily from non-linguistic causes.

Stories are in relation to speaking and hearing what images are to visual perception because the balancing act between finding and inventing that is characteristic for narratives is structurally similar to the paradoxical figure

[33]Taylor develops his argumentation in the confrontation with Harry Frankfurt's claims about reflexive wishing and second order desires. His examples show the constitutive function of the vocabulary used for evaluative, reflected action and the way self-interpretation and experience are mutually conditioned: "self-interpretations are partly constitutive of our experience" (Taylor 2010, p. 37).

of a simultaneously constitutive and responsive force of configuration that is inherent to perception.

2.4 *Visual Culture Studies*

It would be natural to expect a study on the practice of seeing to belong among those hybrid forms of the humanities grouped together in the English-speaking world under the label 'Visual Culture Studies.' This expectation is justified. As demonstrated by the anthologies by Foster (1988), Bryson (1994), Jencks (1995), and Nelson (2000),[34] to name just a few, this discipline has shed light on a broad spectrum of possibilities for seeing and its social, cultural and historical conditions. A good overview is provided in the recent volume by N. Mirzoeff (1999).

Many of these examinations are devoted to the exercise of power through dominant patterns of perception, to the social character of perceptual conventions,[35] and to the environment of the observer,[36] often with the critical intent of revealing the strategies and manipulative interests behind mass media and its inherent sexism and racism.

Another common denominator of this social-pragmatic reconstruction of seeing is the focus on the historical transformation to the status of the seeing subject. In his studies of seeing in the nineteenth century, J. Crary demonstrates perception as an act of attention by which a subject maintains a coherent idea of the world. The conception of the world in turn effects changes in the observer: "an immense social remaking of the observer in the nineteenth century proceeds on the general assumption that perception cannot be thought of in terms of immediacy, presence, punctuality" (Crary 2001, p. 4). Chris Jencks arrives at the same conclusion: "The idea of vision as socially constructed or culturally located both liberates and subsequently elevates the practising 'see-er,' the human actor, from the status of the messenger of nature to the status of theoretician" (Jenks 1995, p. 10).

[34]Nelson's suggestion that visuality is to vision what sexuality is to sex (the former socially, the latter biologically) drags soul–body dualism back into the debate. Hal Foster (1988) denounced this split into the nature and culture of seeing back in 1988.

[35]In this context, Dieter Hoffman-Axthelm's (1984) study is also relevant as a visual culture reading.

[36]Hans Dieter Huber's (2004) investigation strikes a good balance between the appropriate consideration of environmental conditions and internal iconic and aesthetic factors.

These ideas can certainly be usefully adapted if perception is not to be qualified as merely epistemically relevant recognisance. Many of these studies agree with the present book's basic claim that seeing is a culturally conditioned activity and that the visual character of a culture cannot be subsumed under speech and text.[37] However, whereas Visual Culture Studies broadens the field of the visible by focusing on the socio-historical and technological development of instruments and media,[38] the present book is centred on the ethical and aesthetic dimensions of perceptual practice and aspires to put forward insights into art theory and the philosophy of morals.

References

Abel, Günter. 1993. *Interpretationswelten*. Frankfurt am Main: Suhrkamp.

Angehrn, Emil. 2003. *Interpretation und Dekonstruktion*. Weilerswist: Velbrück.

Arendt, Hannah. 1959. *The Human Condition*. Chicago: University of Chicago Press.

Armstrong, David M. 1961. *Perception and the Physical World*. London: Humanities Press.

Austin, John Langshaw. 1962. *Sense and Sensibilia*. Oxford: Oxford University Press.

Ayer, Alfred. 1940. *The Foundation of Empirical Knowledge*. London: Macmillan.

Berkeley, George. 1948. *The Works of George Berkeley, Vol. 1: Philosophical Commentaries—Essay Towards a New Theory of Vision*. London: Nelson.

Böhme, Gernot. 2000. *Platons theoretische Philosophie*. Stuttgart: Metzler.

Brandt, Reinhard. 1999. *Die Wirklichkeit des Bildes*. Munich: Hanser.

Bryson, Norman, Ann Holly, Michael, and Moxey, Keith (ed.). 1994. *Visual Culture: Images and Interpretations*. Middletown: Wesleyan University Press.

Cassirer, Ernst. 1957. *The Philosophy of Symbolic Forms, Volume Three: The Phenomenology of Knowledge*. New Haven: Yale University Press.

Cassirer, Ernst. 1962. *An Essay on Man: An Introduction in the Philosophy of Human Culture*. New Haven: Yale University Press.

Chisholm, Roderick. 1957. *Perceiving*. Ithaca: Cornell University Press.

Condillac, Étienne Bonnot de. 1754. *Traité des sensations*. Paris: De Bure, l'aine.

[37] This is not the place to pit the omnipresence of images in our culture against the dominant text paradigm. Such polemic polarisation is superfluous and indeed counter-productive since it is conditioned by what it attempts to resist.

[38] Jonathan Crary's (1992) study, is one such example of an examination of the technical-practical. It shows how, in the nineteenth century, geometrical optics were replaced by physiological optics and explores the effects this technical innovation had on the role of the observer.

Crary, Jonathan. 1988. Modernizing Vision. In *Vision and Visuality*, ed. Hal Foster, 29–49. Seattle: Bay Press.
Crary, Jonathan. 1992. *Techniques of the Observer*. Cambridge: MIT Press.
Crary, Jonathan. 2001. *Suspensions of Perception: Attention, Spectacle, and Modern Culture*. Cambridge: MIT Press.
Dennett, Daniel. 1991. *Consciousness Explained*. Boston: Little Brown.
Drechsler, Martin. 1995. Sinnesdaten. In *Historisches Wörterbuch der Philosophie*, Bd. 9, Columns 875–882, ed. Joachim Ritter et al. Basel: Schwabe.
Dretske, Fred. 1969. *Seeing and Knowing*. London: Routledge.
Fiedler, Konrad. 1991. *Schriften zur Kunst*. Munich: Fink.
Fodor, Jerry. 1990. Observation Reconsidered. In *A Theory of Content and Other Essays*, 231–251. Cambridge: MIT Press.
Foster, Hal (ed.). 1988. *Vision and Visuality*. Seattle: Bay Press.
Foucault, Michel. 1995. *Discipline and Punish: The Birth of the Prison*. New York: Vintage Books.
Gabriel, Gottfried. 1997. Logisches und analogisches Denken. In *Sprache und Denken*, ed. Alex Burri, 370–384. Berlin: De Gruyter.
Gadamer, Hans-Georg. 2006. *Truth and Method*. London: Bloomsbury Academic.
Gombrich, Ernst. 1960. *Art and Illusion*. Princeton: Princeton University Press.
Goodman, Nelson. 1976. *Languages of Art: An Approach to a Theory of Symbols*. Indianapolis: Bobbs-Merrill.
Goodman, Nelson. 1978. *Ways of Worldmaking*. Indianapolis: Bobbs-Merrill.
Grice, Paul. 1957. Meaning. *The Philosophical Review* 64: 377–388.
Hauschild, Thomas. 1982. *Der Böse Blick*. Berlin: Verlag Mensch und Leben.
Heidegger, Martin. 1996. *Being and Time*. Albany: State University of New York Press.
Hoffman-Axthelm, Dieter. 1984. *Sinnesarbeit*. Frankfurt am Main: Campus.
Hubel, David. 1988. *Eye, Brain, and Vision*. New York: W. H. Freeman & Co.
Huber, Hans Dieter. 2004. *Bild, Beobachter, Milieu*. Ostfildern: Hatje Cantz.
Irigaray, Luce. 1985. *This Sex Which Is Not One*. Ithaca: Cornell University Press.
Irigaray, Luce. 1987. *Speculum of the Other Woman*. Ithaca: Cornell University Press.
James, William. 1950. *The Principles of Psychology*. New York: Dover Publications.
Jay, Martin. 1993. *Downcast Eyes*. Berkeley: University of California Press.
Jencks, Christ. 1995. The Centrality of the Eye in Western Culture. In *Visual Culture*, 1–25. London: Routledge.
Jonas, Hans. 1954. The nobility of sight. *Philosophy and Phenomenological Research* 14 (4): 507–519.
Köhler, Wolfgang. 1969. *The Task of Gestalt Psychology*. Princeton: Princeton University Press.
Kompridis, Nikolas. 1993. Über Welterschließung. *Deutsche Zeitschrift Für Philosophie* 41 (3): 525–538.

Konersmann, Ralf. 1995. Sehen. In *Historisches Wörterbuch der Philosophie Bd. 9*, ed. Joachim Ritter et al., columns 121–161, Basel: Schwabe.
Konersmann, Ralf. 1997. Die Augen der Philosophen. In *Kritik des Sehens*, 9–47. Leipzig: Reclam.
Krämer, Sybille. 2003. Was tut Austin, indem er über das Performative spricht? In *Performativität und Praxis*, ed. Jens Kertscher et al., 19–33. Munich: Fink.
Krämer, Sybille. 2001. *Sprache, Sprechakt, Kommunikation*. Frankfurt am Main: Suhrkamp.
Künne, Wolfgang. 1995. Sehen. Eine Sprachanalytische Betrachtung. *Logos* 2: 103–121.
Langer, Susanne K. 1979. *Philosophy in a New Key: A Study in the Symbolism of Reason, Rite, and Art*. Cambridge: Harvard University Press.
Levin, David (ed.). 1993. *Modernity and the Hegemony of Vision*. Berkeley: University of California Press.
Locke, John. 1975. *An essay Concerning Human Understanding*. Oxford: Oxford University Press.
MacIntyre, Alasdair. 2007. *After Virtue: A Study in Moral Theory*. Notre Dame: University of Notre Dame Press.
Majetschak, Stefan. 1989. Welt als Begriff und Welt als Kunst. *Philosophisches Jahrbuch* 96: 276–293.
McDowell, John. 1994. *Mind and World*. Cambridge: Harvard University Press.
Merleau-Ponty, Maurice. 1962. *Phenomenology of Perception*. London: Routledge.
Mirzoeff, Nicholas (ed.). 1999. *An Introduction to Visual Culture*. London: Taylor & Francis.
Moore, George Edward. 1953. *Some Main Problems of Philosophy*. London: George Allen & Unwin Ltd.
Nelson, R. (ed.). 2000. *Visuality Before and Beyond the Renaissance: Seeing as Others Saw*. Cambridge: Cambridge University Press.
Orth, Ernst Wolfgang. 1992. Ernst Cassirers Philosophie der symbolischen Formen und ihre Bedeutung für unsere Gegenwart. *Deutsche Zeitschrift Für Philosophie* 40 (1/2): 119–136.
Plümacher, Martina. 2004. *Wahrnehmung, Repräsentation und Wissen*. Berlin: Parerga.
Quine, Willard Van Orman. 1953a. On What There Is. In *From a Logical Point of View*, 1–19. Cambridge: Harvard University Press.
Quine, Willard Van Orman. 1953b. Two Dogmas of Empiricism. In *From a Logical Point of View*, 21–46. Cambridge: Harvard University Press.
Recki, Birgit. 2004. *Kultur als Praxis*. Berlin: De Gruyter.
Ricœur, Paul. 1984, 1985, 1988. *Time and Narrative*, 3 vols. Chicago: University of Chicago Press.
Rock, Irvin. 1985. *The Logic of Perception*. New York: MIT Press.
Rorty, Richard. 1989. *Contingency, Irony, and Solidarity*. Cambridge: Harvard University Press.

Rorty, Richard. 1998. Robert Brandom on Social Practices and Representations. In *Truth and Progress, Philosophical Papers, Volume 3*, 122–137. Cambridge: Cambridge University Press.
Ruskin, John. 1858. *The Elements of Drawing*. London: Smith, Elder & Co.
Schildknecht, Christiane. 1999. *Aspekte des Nichtpropositionalen*. Bonn: Bouvier.
Schildknecht, Christiane. 2003. Anschauungen ohne Begriffe? *Deutsche Zeitschrift Für Philosophie* 51: 459–475.
Schumacher, Ralph. 2004. Die kognitive Undurchdringbarkeit optischer Täuschungen. George Berkeleys Theorie visueller Wahrnehmung im Kontext neuerer Ansätze. *Zeitschrift für philosophische Forschung* 58.4: 505–525.
Schwemmer, Oswald. 1997. *Ernst Cassirer*. Berlin: De Gruyter.
Searle, John. 1983. *Intentionality: An Essay in the Philosophy of Mind*. Cambridge: Cambridge University Press.
Seel, Martin. 2004. *Aesthetics of Appearing*. Stanford: Stanford University Press.
Seel, Martin. 2002. Über Richtigkeit und Wahrheit. In *Sich bestimmen lassen*, 45–67. Frankfurt am Main: Suhrkamp.
Sellars, Wilfrid. 1956. *Empiricism and the Philosophy of Mind*. Cambridge: Harvard Press.
Silverman, Kaja. 1997. Dem Blickregime begegnen. In *Privileg Blick*, ed. Christian Kravagna, 41–64. Berlin: Id-Verlag.
Simon, Gérard. 1992. *Der Blick, das Sein und die Erscheinung in der antiken Optik*. Munich: Fink.
Simon, Josef, and Stegmaier, Werner (ed.). 1994. *Zeichen und Interpretation*, 4 Vols. Frankfurt am Main: Suhrkamp.
Singer, Wolf. 2005. Das Bild im Kopf – aus neurobiologischer Perspektive. In *Sichtweisen*, ed. Bernhard Graf et al., 143–160. Wiesbaden: Verlag für Sozialwissenschaften.
Strawson, Peter. 1979. Perception and its Objects. In *Perception and Identity*, ed. Graham F. Macdonald, 41–60. London: Macmillan.
Taylor, Charles. 1985. Self-Interpreting Animals. In *Human Agency and Language*, 45–76. Cambridge: Cambridge University Press.
Taylor, Charles. 2010. What Is Agency? In *Philosophical Papers: Human Agency and Language*, Vol. 1, 15–44. Cambridge: Cambridge University Press.
Thomä, Dieter. 1998. *Erzähle Dich selbst*. Munich: Beck.
Welsch, Wolfgang. 2000. Hegel und die analytische Philosophie. *Information Philosophie* 1: 7–23.
Wiesing, Lambert (ed.). 2002. *Philosophie der Wahrnehmung*. Suhrkamp: Frankfurt am Main.

CHAPTER 3

The Practice of Seeing

A driver sees a red light. A physician inspects a swollen foot. A voyeur spies through a keyhole and is caught in the act. A visitor in a museum is immersed in the observation of a picture. Lovers gaze at each other. All these particular cases of visual perception cannot be subsumed under a general concept without losing their specific characteristics. Absently gazing out of a window, apparently without grasping anything, and the interested look that focuses and identifies are practically opposed to each other among the multitude of possible uses of sight. When is seeing an act of exclusion and selection? When is it a process of completion and when appresentation?[1] What is the type of seeing that involves looking at someone so as to make them uncomfortable or looking at them reproachfully? Seeing clearly encompasses a broad spectrum of actions, from deliberate observation to distracted gliding to communication. Many internal nuances are needed in order to conceptually grasp the different types of visual perception. Further, the activity of seeing is always embedded in social contexts that co-determine its meaning.

The paradigm of seeing as a cognitive identification of the objective world neglects this multiplicity of usages. We quickly reach the limits of the epistemic conception of seeing when we ask, with Wittgenstein, whether it is really possible to *see* sadness or colours or similarity as though they

[1] Husserl's term 'appresentation' refers to the intentional presentation of other possible perceptions, which is added to all perception (see Husserl 1999).

E. Schuermann, *Seeing as Practice*, Performance Philosophy,
https://doi.org/10.1007/978-3-030-14507-1_3

were objects (Wittgenstein 1986, p. 209). It makes a difference whether I am observing a face or a panorama, whether I am looking for my seat in the theatre or giving someone an encouraging look. Such differences are differences of usage and the uses of seeing are as manifold as types of language use. Yet if meaning is a question of usage, nothing tells us that this usage is restricted to following conventional rules. If the use of seeing is not strictly conventional, then an element of variation is inevitably introduced, of creative and individual difference that is contingent on personal conditions. This individual way of seeing can be called the *style of seeing*. The performance of acts of seeing—this much can be presupposed here—is not a stylistically neutral process of taking in what is there.

In looking at someone meaningfully or contemptuously, seeing is an act of interpersonal communication. As such, it belongs to the social world and can generate practical changes within that world. On the other hand, looking out the window and seeing a landscape divided into foreground and background is an activity of perceiving more akin to an act of *configuration*, operating a synthesis of disparate units of information. This synthesis, organising a manifold into a meaningful whole, goes beyond mere *assertion*—that is, noting that such and such is the case.

Nothing of this sort implies knowledge in any relevant form. Seeing images, persons, events, situations and processes are all categorically distinct activities—the performance of which is essentially practical—that involve tasks that cannot be entirely assimilated to epistemic acts. With the aid of the concept of practice, it should be possible to grasp seeing as an individualised act of attention rooted simultaneously in social and interpersonal practice.

Practice does not follow an anonymous procedure but is co-shaped by individual agents, i.e. perceivers whose perspectives manifest in collective stereotypes and in individual differences. Performance is a basic constituent of practice that needs to be looked at in more detail later. The culturally and personally conditioned blind spots and gradations[2] that make seeing so variegated would seem to issue from the active character of visual attention as something performed—that is, carried out. It is the performance of perception that determines individually what is seen and how. However, before looking at the question of performance, we must first work out other implications of the concept of practice.

[2]On the concept of gradations [*Abschattungen*; literally: shades] (see Husserl 1997).

1 Shared Visibility

In philosophy, practice generally denotes a network of interdependent activities. In the context of a practice, agents, speakers and perceivers are parts of a web of framing conditions, which are not ready-made in the manner of unequivocal, predicable objects but are developed by the forms of life of a culture and an epoch, by the language use of a respective community and by social norms. Practice is a set of relations between interpersonal activities and their structural preconditions. The essential feature of these conditions is that meaning is collectively negotiated and generated within a shared world. Meaning is thus intersubjective and interactive and can be cooperative or conflictual. As such, 'accurate perception' is subject to intersubjective examination and social authorisation. Grasping seeing as practice means becoming aware of the social and historical contingencies that enable and distort the individual's vision.

In the Kantian version, practice is what is made possible by the exercise of freedom (see Kant 1998, p. 674). It can therefore be assumed at this juncture that the practice of seeing is perhaps realised in one's freedom to see in different ways, in the ability of seeing to interpret and reinterpret. This power is restricted in its movement by the social regulation of practice as by a gravitational pull.

1.1 The Logic of Practice

Among modern theories of practice, that of Pierre Bourdieu (1990, 1991, 1998) can be usefully applied to explain practice as the active, situated means of relating to others and relating with others to a mutually inhabited world in ways that are constrained by historical, social and cultural horizons. Bourdieu sets himself off from instrumentalistic and intentionalistic notions of action when examining the logic of practice. He demonstrates that practice, as opposed to observation as a theoretical comportment, presupposes specific involvement in a self-sufficient practical order and its temporal dynamics, which are not visible to the agents in the way objects are. According to Bourdieu, "performative Practice […] strives to bring about what it acts or says" (Bourdieu 1990, p. 92), i.e. practice is a field of actions that cannot be described by the model of tool use, because this would presuppose both the tool and the reality in a pregiven form, whereas performative action generates what it performs by performing it.

Bourdieu's theory of practice is interesting both in terms of content and method. He opposes both substantialistical description, which hypostatises the constitutive factors in practice into mutually external and independent entities. He introduces a 'first principle of relations,' describing the connection between objective structures of social space (the field) and the embodied dispositions of the agents (habitus) as a generative web of relations. His aim is to develop a concept of practice that avoids reifying both the structures and the agents. This concept is to take account of the unavoidable institutional and socio-economic contingencies of practice, without thereby reducing the agents thus conditioned to "mere epiphenomenal manifestations of the structure" (Bourdieu 1998, p. 41).

The field referred to is the institutionalised social and historical order, which provides the basic structural conditions of possible action and is at once generated by the collective contributions of all the agents, often via conflict. The agents' particular habitus is their individual and supra-individual way of speaking, perceiving and acting; or rather their habitus is that individuality of their thinking and acting that they could develop under the conditions of a particular time and placed within a particular social and historical order.

Bourdieu's model of practice can be employed in order to remove seeing beyond the one-sidedness of representation theory. The model's virtue is that it helps to undermine the objectivist notion of a disjunction between a subject and an object. Following Bourdieu's model, vision can also be released from the false dichotomy between autonomous construction and passive reflection. Seeing can thus be described as a way of relating to the world within practice, subject to a series of external influences and constituted jointly by the collective and the individual.

1.2 *The Field of Practice*

Merleau-Ponty develops his concept of practice as a network of independent conditions within which the agent and the acts, the subject and objects, are inseparably interwoven. "The profound philosophical meaning of the notion of practice is to place us in an order that is not that of knowledge but rather that of communication, exchange and association" (Merleau-Ponty 1973, p. 50). The emphasis here is less on the institutional and social framework conditioning practice than on its anchoring in that which the author explains as bodily being-in-the-world. Merleau-Ponty also formulates a field theory of practice in which agents are compared with players on a playing field. "For the player in action the football field is not an 'object' [...] It is pervaded with lines of force [...] which call for a certain mode of action [...] as if the player were unaware of it. The field itself is not given to him, but present as the immanent term of his practical intentions; the player becomes one with it and feels the direction of the 'goal,' for example, just as immediately as the vertical and the horizontal planes of his own body" (Merleau-Ponty 2004, p. 53).

Accordingly, intersubjective practice is shaped by the dynamics of a *field formation* that is prefigured in the body. Here. the field supplies a further figure of speech for describing the relations of the participating agents with other factors without recourse to subject–object terminology. The relations are neither subjective in the sense of free, arbitrary constructions, nor objective in the sense of substantial, pre-existent entities. Rules of play restrain arbitrariness in the practice, which is thereby determined neither by mere private constructions nor by objective givens.

In what follows, the term practice will be used in the sense mentioned above. A different descriptive language is required to free the understanding of the practice of perception from objectivist thinking. The practice theories of Bourdieu and Merleau-Ponty provide a vocabulary for considering the viewer and the visible as a network of interdependencies, which is more appropriate than the categories of subject and object.

2 Seeing as Doing

Just as the performance of speech acts creates or alters reality, so too can seeing occasion practical effects. It is this fact that authorises the assertion that seeing is doing. Although the efficacy of seeing usually consists in predication and identification, it can also include the freedom to *revise*, *review* and to see differently as well as involving productive ruptures in the ordinary conventions of seeing. Seeing is an activity that involves dealing with the polyvalence of the visible world.

The practical dimension is not merely an accidental trait applying to special cases of perception, but rather a fundamental structural feature common to all forms of perception. It must be presupposed as a logical constituent of vision together with the viewer and the visible. Just as any practice can be both active and reactive, so too does seeing—understood as an activity—oblige us to react to the way that the visible world is socially configured and thereby to respond to it in the sense of response indicated by Arendt. Just as intermissive practice is a form of activity, so too does a passive, inattentive 'seeing that' leave the visible to its own devices; rather than appropriating it, it remains a kind of activity. As a dimension of practice, seeing encompasses the possibilities of both determining and being determined.[3] As such, seeing can never be an arbitrary act of construction, but is rather an act of constitution involving mediation.

To further expand on the comparison with speech act theory, it can be shown that Austin's distinction between locutionary, illocutionary and perlocutionary (Austin 1975, see especially Lecture 8) speech acts can also be applied to vision. Seeing-*something* and seeing-*that* occur more or less on a level comparable to the locutionary level. One operates on the illocutionary level by doing something in a more targeted way; for example, by finding something or getting in touch with someone. Such activities necessarily have perlocutionary effects on the person being looked at and on our immediate world generally.

The common distinction in semiotics between syntax, semantics and pragmatics pushes the issue a step further.[4] The difference between a syntactic and a semantic orientation is present both in acts of vision and in speech acts. Various constituent elements of the process of perception can be distinguished with its aid: Such elements of the act of seeing condition the way a copy or mirror-like function of seeing relates to its interpretive components, how partial and holistic seeing mutually determine each other and how a panoramic overview misses details. Depending on whether perception is concentrated more on the formal features of the thing seen or on possible semantic determinants, it becomes a different kind of act, contributing in varying degrees to the constitution of the larger event of which it is a part.

It is difficult to bring systematic unity to the various processes of differentiation, organisation, shape making, selection, filtering, pattern constitution and schematising. A few basic principles can, however, be identified.

[3]Martin Seel has explained this connection between doing and letting be in connection with his notion of self-determination, showing that a conscious and definite decision is often a decision to let oneself be determined from the outside (Seel 2002, pp. 279–298, especially 289f.). For the theory of practice, this duplicity is crucial to escape dichotomies such as that of active and autonomous vs. passive and heteronymous. The same must be shown for the practice of perception.

[4]Charles W. Morris (1970) originally introduced this distinction for application to all sign use. It has since become autonomous and has demonstrated its elucidative power in numerous contexts.

2.1 Syntactic Seeing How

When we see in terms of form, light, shade, magnitude, depth, mass and proportion, we are concerned with the formal structural elements of the visible world. Just as the syntax of a sentence is based on a general set of rules, so too is the visible based on basic structures, on depth, relations, surfaces, contours and so on. The optical presence of objects is organised by values of visibility in a way that is comparable to the organisation of sentence structure. Forms, colours, directionality, and masses constitute a kind of grammar of seeing. By strengthening or dissolving contrasts, perception differentiates a multitude of visual information into an organised unity.[5] If seeing were an arbitrary collection of unrelated visual data, the coherent perception of gestalt would necessarily be a procedure distinct from it. Gestalt psychology has demonstrated the ordering power of visual perception. We do not perceive chaos, but rather meaningful sets of relations. Seeing exhibits an order-generating capacity by which it discloses the structure and appearance of the external world. Seeing the whole involves more than adding up individual parts. Dynamic formal qualities, suggestive impressions, contrasts, the tectonic structure of the visible, its expressive gestalt qualities and the spatial network of relations of which the visible is part are configured synoptically. Gestalt perceptions, the sharpening of contour, recognising prominent [prägnant] forms,[6] all of these take place on a quasi-syntactic level. Arnold Gehlen referred to the ability to form and isolate gestalt out of perceptions as '*Prägnanztendenz*' [the tendency toward meaningfulness] (Gehlen 1966, part two, §16, pp. 157–180, 158). This is not to be confused with the nineteenth century 'sensation atomism' familiar from William James and the early gestalt theorists.[7] Instead, it is a synthetic power to perceive coherence.

What Heidegger called "the specific 'syn' character of pure intuition" (Heidegger 1962, p. 152), begins with the capacity of seeing to make separations and connections. Seeing unities and differences is not the same as *making distinctions*, which is characteristic for an 'observer' in Luhmann's

[5] A wealth of clearly organised examples can be found in R. S. Crutchfield (1982).

[6] A gestalt is 'prägnant' in psychology of perception when its simplicity generates visual preferences. (Goldstein 2002). An excellent overview of insights from gestalt theory regarding visual arts is provided by Max J. Kobbert (1982).

[7] A good overview of the work by Ehrenfels, Metzger and Köhler is provided by M. Wertheimer (1974).

sense. It is instead the recognition of differences within a coherent whole. It is not a conceptual operation, but rather an act of perceptual structuring and integration in dealing with contrasts, proportions, surfaces, reliefs, gestalts and distances.

Pure concentration on such parameters of visibility is rare in everyday life. However, there will be few cases where syntactic seeing is altogether absent since it is the basis of all cognitive vision. I see a fir tree by means of a vertical thrust, dark colours and a silhouette tapering to a point. As long as I desist from reflecting on the fact that these designations belong to the fir tree, the semantic identity of what I am looking at remains uncertain and I see only its visual structure. I see syntactically when I do not attribute meaning, perceiving only the way it is visible, the *how* of its visibility.

In the chapter *Seeing art*, it will be shown that we must assume a layer to vision prior to social figuration in order to describe the painting of Cézanne. On this syntactic level, seeing is indifferent to meaning, giving voice to a 'pre-propositional' language of the visible. Paying attention to the modality by which something is made visible reveals something that remains concealed to the type of seeing concerned, above all, with identifying objects. It leads not to secure knowledge but at best to knowledge by acquaintance. It abstracts from the *what* of the object seen, blocking out the general knowledge of the object that allows it to be classified in favour of attentive observation of how it presents itself in a particular light from a particular perspective in a particular setting. This type of seeing is syntactic to the extent that it overlooks practically all of the habitual meanings attached to the thing seen.

2.2 Semantic Seeing As

The syntactic act of seeing must be principally distinguished from a mode of seeing concerned with discovering and attributing meaning, with understanding and interpreting. The systematic intertwinement of sight and insight, interpretation and understanding, will be explored in more depth later. For the time being, we will concern ourselves with a provisional set of logical distinctions.

Seeing a fir tree as a fir tree is to be distinguished from seeing a dark, tapered silhouette by the semantic identification of the form being seen as a tree of this type. In our terminology, all cognitive seeing that identifies or classifies the Seen is semantic. We have, however, established that cognitive *seeing-that* need not be intentional. Semantic *seeing-something-as-something* can occasionally go far beyond the epistemic, when it imaginatively invents meaning; for example, by seeing figures in clouds or in a Rorschach test. Seeing the cloud *as* an elephant tends more to invention than to 'recognition.' To see forms in the amorphous is to generate a meaning, the existence of which is due in equal parts to perception and to imagination. It would be reductive to subsume the inventive, productive quality of seeing under the epistemic paradigm.

On the semantic level, seeing becomes a procedure of articulation and configuration that reaches beyond cognition, receiving significant contributions from emotions, desires, empathy and imagination.

Another example of this possible use of seeing is seeing *that* someone is something. In order to see, for example, that someone is bothered by something, seeing must be endowed with a capacity to constitute sense. This capacity, although occasioned by sensibility, is inexplicable in sensualist terms. Seeing that someone is distracted is literally to *see* something, rather than hearing, touching or simply imagining it without any sensory occasion to do so.[8] Thought and interpretation still play a constitutive roll in this type of seeing, which is the reason why it is possible to attribute the wrong meaning.

Talk of attributing meaning can be misleading. Designating this type of seeing as basically neuro-physiological stimulus-reaction plus posterior generation of meaning would be a regression into the myth of the innocent eye. When we come to Wittgenstein's aspect-seeing, it will become clear that seeing as a semantic practice is an exemplary case of the inseparability of perception and interpretation. In seeing something *as* something, the act of judgement is not added on afterwards, but occurs simultaneously with the visual act of disclosure. I do not first see something and then tend to consider it under this or that aspect. I instantaneously see this or that thing.

Intentional seeing-something-as-something under the gradually variable participation of the imagination is to be understood as a semantic visual practice. There is a higher degree of imaginative interpretation than in the syntactic *seeing of form* and classificatory *seeing of objects*, because it involves the participation of a 'will to see' that is more than a mere state of wishing.

[8]The same goes for hearing; for example, hearing on the telephone that someone is embarrassed by a question. The structure is the same: something is both found as pre-existing and disclosed within sensory perception.

This will must be regarded, as it is by Wittgenstein, as part of the action itself.[9] Semantic seeing is the inventive constitution of a mode of vision that operates not by granting direct access to a definite pre-existent entity but rather by opening an iconic type of mediation between the self and the world.

2.3 *Pragmatic and Practical Seeing*

It will be useful at this stage to consider the practical character of seeing in terms of a pragmatic-purposive side and a practical-ethical side. Vision can be regarded as pragmatic when it serves as a means to an end in dealing with the demands of living. Seeing as practice involves more—namely, it is a moral way of disclosing a world that is perceivable to the senses and socially shared. Common to both aspects is the dimension of action. Seeing is in both cases an active way of functioning within the world of social visibility.

Consequently, other people are no less fundamental to understanding the practice of perception than the person doing the seeing. To the extent that seeing is a practice, it is related to others. 'You,' 'us,' and 'them' are present to seeing even when they are physically absent. Being publicly visible makes seeing a practical affair with social ramifications. This not only implies a dyadic relation to other particular individuals implicated in the ramifications of interpersonal visibility; in equal measure, it involves the generalised, internalised *other* as instantiated by society and the milieu. G. H. Mead described these processes with the distinction between 'me' and 'I' (Mead 1992). 'Me' is the self as an object mirrored back to the 'I' in the eyes of the others. 'I' is the synthetic identity of these many 'mes,' a consistent self-image. 'Me' is identity from the perspective of the others. It is constituted by means of normativity, evaluation and narrative. The self constitutes its identity by perceiving the perceptions others make of it, by mediating between 'I' and 'me,' or by bringing them into mutual agreement. Like Fichte's 'I,' which always only grasps its object-I, while never grasping itself as subject-I, so too is Mead's 'I' "a fictitious 'I' always out of sight of itself" (Mead 1912, p. 406). For all that, it has nevertheless

[9] "Willing, if it is not to be a sort of wishing, must be the action itself. It cannot be allowed to stop anywhere short of the action. If it is the action, then it is so in the ordinary sense of the word; so it is speaking, writing, walking, lifting a thing, imagining something. But it is also trying, attempting, making an effort, to speak, to write, to lift a thing, to imagine something etc" (Wittgenstein 1986, p. 160).

internalised all the more the gazes of its fellow humans. The generalised *other* constitutes the *other* in the self. A self constitutes consciousness of itself by what it is, was or seems to be in the eyes of the others. This is not metaphorical talk, but an anthropological *Existential.* Concrete bodily visibility is the condition of social visibility. This will be explained in more detail further on in the book. It should suffice in the meantime to hold onto the notion that the shared living community, with its beliefs, demands, interests and conventions, is constitutive for the way we see ourselves and others.

Seeing as a practice certainly does not change the state of things and affairs in the physical world in the same way as something like chopping wood does.[10] That seeing is an activity does not imply that the material stock of the world is increased by the addition of new objects or that pre-existent material is altered. However, seeing is a means of effecting changes in the social world; for example, by the use of speech. The communicative effects that a meaningful look, be it admiring or reproachful, has on the person being looked at, can, under certain circumstances, permanently alter that person's psychological state. By affecting relations of mutual acknowledgement, interpersonal seeing changes the self-relation of the person seen. Experiences of seeing and being seen are thus part of the process of personal development. In the same way as the execution of speech acts creates and changes realities, perceptual realities are constituted and altered in and by seeing.

3 Worlds of Perception

In the following, a heuristic distinction will be drawn within the various usages of seeing between instrumental (means to an end) and self-purposive (end in itself) activities. Since Aristotle, practice has been divided into the poietic and the practical, making and doing, whereby making is toward an ulterior purpose and doing is self-purposive: "Included within the class of what can be otherwise are what is produced and what is done. Production and action are different [...] For while production has an end distinct from

[10]Chopping wood is Rüdiger Bubner's example of the altering capacity of an action. Bubner backs into a strangely reductionist argumentation when claiming that the practice of thinking, such as solving the problem of transcendental deduction, does not change the world whereas chopping wood does (Bubner 1976, p. 76). The present book does not presuppose this type of materialist understanding of what alteration could mean.

itself, this could not be so with action, since the end here is acting well itself" (Aristotle 2000, 1140a and 1140b).[11] Accordingly, poiesis is the production of an Εργον, praxis is Ενργεια, whose purpose is ipso actu. In other words, *making* is the production of a work, and *practice* is action whose purpose is in itself.

Language use can be the means to the end of information and communication, yet language and speech go beyond this to include Ενργεια, which fulfils itself in the doing, as Humboldt in particular has clearly demonstrated (Humboldt 1973, p. 36f.). By the same token, the deployment of the sense of sight must be divided into an instrumental and a self-purposive side. What has above been described as epistemic seeing is largely a poietic activity, the purpose of which is external to itself—that is, in the resulting identification of objects in the world. As in speech, the Εργον is in this case not a thing but a result in which the purpose of activity is fulfilled. Everyday perception for the purpose of providing orientation in the world and coping with practical challenges is an instrumental activity in that ends are intended and effected by it, to which end seeing is the appropriate means.

This type of seeing needs to be distinguished from seeing that attains its end in the performance itself. In the latter case, the means *are* the end, the meaning of perception is realised in the act, without recourse to a tangible ulterior result. In Hannah Arendt's reading of the Aristotelian notion, actual activities are those "that do not pursue an end [...] and leave no work behind [...], but exhaust their full meaning in the performance itself" (Arendt 1958, p. 206). Cases of casual, disinterested, wandering gazing are familiar examples from everyday life where seeing takes on the character of a non-intentional, medial encounter between someone seeing and something seen.

I will apply this distinction between Εργον and Ενργεια, medium and mediality, means and end, to three different areas: seeing everyday objects; the aesthetic seeing of images and presentations; and the ethical seeing of persons.

Everyday seeing can be construed largely though not entirely within an epistemic paradigm. In the case of interpersonal seeing and being seen, the most interesting aspect is the existential significance of being visible in the gaze of the other, with all its ramifications for interpersonal acknowledgement, identity constitution and communication. In the case of seeing art,

[11] See also idem (2008, 1048b).

the main focus is on the interferences between perception and imagination and the semantic characteristics of aisthesis. We practice perception within different practical situations entailing the presentation of different worlds. The world of art requires and enables other practices than those found in everyday life, the world of intersubjectivity other qualities than those used in the sciences. General cases of perceptual practice can be differentiated according to their functions in everyday life, in aesthetics and in ethics for the sole reason that each of these perceptual worlds is "a made reality" (Arendt 1958, p. 288)—that is, not given in the manner of a substance but rather as a complex situation constituted by practice.

The attempt to emphasise the dominant characteristics and the qualitative uniqueness of each form of seeing inevitably leads to a somewhat artificial stylising of the three classes of perception as types. The daily encounter with the postman in the morning can be taken as a case of interpersonal communicative seeing, but it is equally certain that this is rarely an instance of strong communication. What will be discussed here as interpersonal, mutual seeing is reserved for ethically significant encounters with other persons.

Since pragmatic everyday seeing has the tendency to be largely purposive, for the sake of avoiding over-complexity, the main focus of this book is on ethically and aesthetically meaningful seeing. Seeing faces and images provides the model for understanding the ethical-aesthetic practice of seeing. The chapters in which this is worked out will demonstrate concretely and in detail how such seeing is a form of performative world disclosure.

The dilemma for any theoretical description of practice is that it necessarily undoes that practice's logic. A conceptual explanation of the practical hybrid forms of perception in intersubjective contexts and everyday living situations cannot avoid making inclusive and exclusive classifications. However, these classifications clearly show how complex the interplay is between the factors involved in the practice of perception. The dynamic totality of a practice eludes the divisions inherent in description. All attempts at theoretical explanation of a practice are confronted with this problem. As Bourdieu asserts, explaining the incommensurability of theoretical explanation and practice, "The shift from the practical scheme to the theoretical schema [...] lets slip everything that makes the temporal reality of practice in process" (Bourdieu 1990, p. 81). Theoretical reflection transposes the progress in time of consecutive and simultaneous individual acts into the order of an illuminated and configured total act and shifts the perspective from the first person to the observer. The person observed is no longer what she was, she becomes something else, because reason and preconditions are claimed that turn the ambivalence and complexity of the practice into something with a single unified meaning.

This need not invalidate all theory. Freed from the pressure of pragmatic forces, theory is supposed to exemplify the "non-limited" (Adorno 1977, p. 477). The following reflections offer primarily a heuristic explication of terms that the subsequent line of argument will bear out more closely.

An entirely different approach is required for the sciences. The scientific gaze is not only a genuine form of exact empirical observation, it is also—furnished with the appropriate technical instruments—the discloser of invisible worlds.[12] However, an important difference emerges here. Scientific seeing is principally concerned with *other forms of invisibility* than ethical and aesthetic seeing. When x-rays render matter transparent, endoscopes illuminate the inside of the body and when the effects of elementary particles are visualised, something is made visible that would have remained invisible without the technical preparation.[13] The case of the moral-practical world is different in that it is also invisible to specialised equipment, since it is the invisibility of the imaginary and ideational, or that of meaning we are concerned with in this context. The first variety of invisibility is imperceptible to non-technically enhanced observation. The other—such as anger in a face or the idea of the infinite in romantic painting—is a sui generis type of invisibility, which will need to be more closely defined in accordance with the ethical-aesthetic focus of the enquiry.

[12]Interesting in this connection is: H. Böhme (2004). Böhme identifies in the history of science and medicine, in particular in seventeenth century vacuum theory, the same paradoxical simultaneity of production and mediation that I am claiming for seeing; a 'performative mediality' as the "mechanism, that in the process of representation creates at the same time as it represents" (ibid., p. 215).

[13]To speak here of technical preparation is more accurate than technical instruments such as microscopy or telescopy. Particle physics, for example, is an interesting rupture with models of scientific seeing based on the human eye, because elementary particles are too fast to be made visible. Telescopic and microscopic seeing are structurally similar to natural seeing, delivering to the eyes very small and very distant things as though they were visible without instruments. This is precisely no longer true of the proofs of particles moving in an accelerator. In contrast to the smallest microscopic particles, elementary particles are no longer visible at all. Only the traces of their effects can be visualised. The preparatory effort required to make them visible is so great that the manipulations involved appear constitutive for the observation of the observed. Therefore, scientific seeing must be seen to be as much a case of creation as discovery.

3.1 Seeing as Means and Seeing as End in Everyday Life

The common meaning of seeing for the purpose of gaining information about visible things, orienting oneself and recognising things and situations can be described—with a pinch of salt—within the epistemic paradigm. Seeing taken as the function of information gathering with the eyes basically boils down to recognisant or cognisant and constative seeing-that. I see whether a picture is hanging straight on the wall by registering states of affairs in the visible world. Checking to see if my shoes are wet, to see the number of books I should pack, checking my bag to see if the keys are there and establishing that the table is brown are all examples of a seeing that has nothing to do with apprehending presence, but can instead be understood as registering and predicating.

The most familiar form of the everyday use of the sense of sight is presumably the attribution and classification of what is directly in front of us. We recognise something we know and is literally "in the picture," we note the things present and their states for the purpose of orientation. By contrast, the examining gaze focuses and discovers, goes into detail, in order to acquire knowledge about the thing seen. Revelations by means of exact, penetrating looking, the gaze capable of seeing behind the facade, are examples of this type of seeing. Forms of *inspection* or exploration [Erkunden], as well as, more positively connoted, *watching over* [Hüten] and *watching out* [Aufpassen] demarcate the field of surveillance, whose relation to power has been subjected to critique since Bentham's panopticon and Foucault's critical analysis of synoptic regimes of the gaze.

However, when not employed as a means to an ulterior end, seeing can develop its character as performance of an act even in practical everyday contexts. Non-intentional seeing, such as gazing out of a train window lost in thought, seeing that relinquishes a determination/identification of what it is seeing, because it is devoted to seeing of the landscape and cities fleeting by; the distracted gaze, meandering over space without particular intent, does not primarily identify, even if it leads to this or that opinion about things and persons in space.

It is probably exigent to presuppose a kind of involuntary, partially pre-reflexive seeing—that is, the reception of fragmentary, aimless impressions, even though this gets dangerously close to the notion of a basic perception. This should not set us back behind our own insights but rather enable us to better distinguish this form of seeing from other forms of seeing. Seeing that apprehends something can thereby be distinguished from acts of evaluation without requiring us to assume an isolatable procedure of sensory stimulus response. Involuntary seeing entails a low degree of interpretation and therefore belongs to the class of casual viewing in everyday contexts. Only a part of the information gleaned by the eyes in seeing reaches consciousness.

The term 'habitual seeing' could be used to refer to something closely related to involuntary seeing. Conventions of seeing are developed over the course of a lifetime and inform what we are used to seeing. Typical forms of no-longer-seeing and overlooking result from this fact. Not everything that seeing leaves out can be explained exclusively by affective or imaginative dispositions but it often is due to behavioural habits of seeing and socially agreed rules. Schematised stereotypes emerge in this way. Without such stereotypes, getting around in life would be overwhelmingly complex. No longer seeing in seeing, an event of vision constituted by a fundamental negativity, is often due in concrete instances to habitual expectation. When someone enters a room where they are used to seeing a piano, the piano is usually no longer perceived in the fullness of its sensory apparition, although it would immediately be noticed if it were missing. What is no-longer-perceived is sufficiently present to echo in every act of vision. The same applies to peripheral vision. We do not consciously see what an object on the far right of our field of vision looks like but we would immediately notice if it moved.

How much of daily seeing is really *seeing* and how much presupposition of the expected and familiar can only be decided in each case. A certain habitus, in Bourdieu's sense of the term, that can develop into a style, referred to by Proust as "a vision"[14] (Proust 1993, p. 299) reveals itself in the way we see habitually and diverge from the habitual seeing of others.

3.2 Seeing as Means and Seeing as End in the Aesthetic

Such cases of perception where the act implies judgements of taste, such as looking at clothing, furniture, choosing fabrics and so on tend to belong to the epistemic function of sight. They are more directed at ends than, say, the contemplation of art engaged in for its own sake, and more similar to the scrutinising gaze of information gathering. The assessing gaze, estimating

[14]This point will be treated at greater length further on.

the monetary value of an artwork, or the expert gaze rapidly ascribing a piece to its époque or a period within the artist's oeuvre, is not aesthetically self-purposive, but rather instrumental.

When a commercial photographer sees, her seeing could be meaningfully qualified as work. If a photo results from this process, one can retrospectively refer to her act as 'making' because an object has arisen from it. For fashion designers, interior designers, decorators, set designers—that is, for people working with the aesthetic appearance of objects, people and situations—seeing is not a continuous act of uncertain duration and direction, but a professional act with an aim and a result.

The gaze of the artist, be it that of a painter, photographer, filmmaker or similar, breaks out of such criteria. This gaze can be regarded as work due to its professional and directed nature, but it also contains just as many self-purposive elements. Each gaze belongs to a certain aesthetic and is committed to a certain style and usually in a specific way that is different to conventional seeing, to which I will return in the chapter on art.

Experiences of presence, which are an end in themselves and are realised in their own achievement, make aesthetic seeing an autonomous act. Seeing here is not an instrument, but rather involves a *letting be* type of awareness, a being addressed by a thing seen. Examples are seeing a sunset or the experience of a view from a mountain summit. Here, seeing does not arrive at a definite result. Instead, the path is the destination. Various forms of optical desire, more involved in pleasure than in reflection, also belong here. G. Böhme has described such seeing as the observer "being-alongside" (Böhme 2000) the observed.[15] When we perceive atmospheres and moods, seeing is more like self-abandonment than assertion. In the bracketing of the usual predicative function of seeing, the aesthetic perception harbours possibilities of seeing 'with other eyes.' This will be explored more closely in Chapter 9.

3.3 Seeing as Means and Seeing as End in the Ethical

I understand the concept of the ethical in the broadest possible sense, subsuming under it all those cases in which other persons play a role whose presence makes perception a determination of social visibility. Those forms of seeing that make this most clear are interpersonal seeing and being seen.

[15] This form of seeing could partly be explained with the adverbial theory of perception, as advocated by C. Ducasse (1951). A helpful commentary is provided in L. Wiesing (2002).

Being concretely visible as a body is an existentially and morally significant event, just as constitutive for building personal identity as for linguistic activity. This problem could be approached from the perspectives of developmental psychology, psychology and psychoanalysis as well as from the point of view of socialisation. For each concept, a notion of the imagination is required, since the ability to put ourselves in another's place, to imaginatively anticipate their standpoints, and to assume roles and absorb social norms all presuppose participation of the imagination in perception.

This section has to do with the concept of practice with the aid of the distinction between self-purposive and instrumental action, means and ends. This will first require indicating why seeing can at all be a moral-practical occasion. Interpersonal seeing and being visible represent a genuine form of perceptual relation to self and world, not least due to the reciprocity of relations of looking, which constitute the core of personhood in seeing.[16] In living together socially, looks are often a means of communication. The communicative employment of the eyes is thus a good example of instrumental seeing in the intersubjective context.

As Sartre has shown (Sartre 1992, pp. 340–401), such seeing can, in certain circumstances, develop an eminently objectifying power. An examination of his theory of the look as a performative act of attribution and development of self-consciousness will demonstrate that the ethical relevance of perceptual practice resides in judgemental, normative ascriptions of identity. Gazing at the other makes her feel caught in the act, subject to surveillance, and degraded to an object for the gaze of others.

The power of the look in the social context, the indifferent sexualised or indiscrete look, the pedagogical look that wordlessly praises and reproves, are all examples of types of look-relations exercising perlocutionary effects on the recipients of the look.

Visual communication possesses a certain kind of eloquence akin to that of language. Looks can be exchanged just as words can be exchanged. A

[16]Although there is an artificial quality to a terminological distinction between *seeing* and *looking at*, it can perhaps be said that looking at tends to relate to seeing as individual actions to practice and speech acts to speech. This means that looking at tends to be a pointed act aimed at a particular address. It has perlocutionary significance and can be deployed as a means, whereas seeing implies the non-conclusive character of practice and speech. Yet of course a look can wander about peripatetically without a particular aim, just as, inversely, seeing guided by interests leads to a tangible result and end beyond itself; that end being the information being sought for. The particularity of the interpersonal look appears to reside in reciprocity. This will be discussed in more detail in Chapter 8, Sect. 1.

look can be perceived as a promise, can make demands or give warnings. This is not merely a metaphorical expression from which a literal meaning could be skimmed off, since the pragmatic consequences are palpable in the physical world. In such cases where people communicate with silent looks and then do something—for instance, get up to dance because they have taken in the appropriate ocular prompts, or they repress an utterance after observing a warning look—seeing is a genuine form of speaking and communicating.

It can of course be objected that such effects are generated not only by seeing but by the context in which seeing is performed. Only in the environment of the dance party or the family celebration can these examples be felt as invitations or warnings. Nevertheless, the dependency on the institutional, conventional and situative contexts worked out by the speech act theory of Austin, Searle and Strawson (see Strawson 1964, pp. 439–460), does not alter the fact that it is an aisthetic act that has relevant effects. Like the institution of marriage, which invests determined speakers with the authority to perform actions with juridical effects by speaking, so too does seeing depend on its practical context in order to realise its character as doing. The speech act and the communicative look are prerequisites for occasioning practical effects.

Austin's concern was partly to demonstrate that sentences are contingent on context and that their meaning results from the use of language within practice (Austin 1961, 1975). The conventionality of this use is "rule governed behaviour" (Searle 1969, p. 17)—that is, the context regulates what can be meant by a word. The conventional use of seeing is due no less to its embeddedness in contexts and forms of life as that of speech acts. The ways seeing can be deployed and understood depend on rules of play in day-to-day practice.

What someone *is* in the public eye [*Öffentlichkeit*; literally: openness], in the concretion as well as in the generalisation of the others, and what is reflected back as self-image conditions a qualitative leap from the self to self-consciousness, thus making seeing an act invested with the power to bestow acknowledgement (Honneth 1996, 2003). The cases of morally significant seeing extend from more or less violent processes of subjectivisation, as described by Foucault and Butler (Butler 1997), to unconditional recognition. As Lévinas has shown in particular (Lévinas 1969), Sartre's version of interpersonal seeing is one-sided, neglecting an indispensable property of this occurrence. A human face cannot be looked at in the same way as a random object. Lévinas'treatment of the gaze and the face is therefore a suitable exemplification of the non-instrumental dimension of the act of seeing persons. For Lévinas, seeing the other entails the acknowledgement of a moral responsibility: "This gaze that supplicates and demands [...] which one recognizes in giving (as one 'puts the things in question in giving')— this gaze is precisely the epiphany of the face as a face" (Lévinas 1969, p. 75). It will be discussed further on in the book to what extent the gaze being referred to here is to be understood literally and empirically. It is, however, in any case concerned with a type of seeing that is difficult to describe as mere visual communication. Looking and being looked at constitute an interpersonal exercise of freedom.

This was probably pointed out first of all by J. G. Fichte. He too takes his point of departure from the concrete physical visibility in the gaze of the other: "My body must be visible to the person outside me; it must appear to him through the medium of light, and it must have appeared to him, as surely as he exercises an efficacy on me" (Fichte 2000, p. 71). The ethical weight this being visible develops in its character as demand[17] is qualified by Fichte as mutual recognition (see Siep 1979; Wildt 1982). The other demands that I make use of my freedom when the way she looks at me involves this appeal. The character of appeal within this occurrence is very similar to what Lévinas describes as the irresistible appeal of the face.

We cannot here embark on the theme of recognition—as reflected by Fichte in his theory of natural right and by Hegel in his Jena-period *Realphilosophie*, the Philosophy of Right and the Encyclopaedia, which was finally historically influential in the master-bondsman chapter of the Phenomenology of Spirit—and engage in all its transcendental-philosophical depth. The question at hand is simply which insights can be drawn from it for the theory of seeing as practice. There is a systematic connection where being physically visible makes concrete the processes of recognition within life. Being seen empirically by the imaginarily intersected gaze of the other is decisive for the development of self-consciousness. It could be objected that this is no longer 'proper' seeing. However, apart from the fact that the assumption of a 'proper seeing' if it refers to a basic physiological stimulus-response, has already proved to be much too problematic, it cannot be denied that social visibility is based on physical visibility in the gaze of the other and is as such more than mere figurative speech. Physical

[17] For further explanations see C. H. Hegemann (1982). See also: E. Düsing (1986).

visibility is to social visibility presumably as sex is to gender. Sex does not occur without gender, which is, however, not perceivable as such.

The meaning of perception for the development of self-consciousness is only realised actively and in the process. Recognition is necessarily active, for which reason Fichte describes it as "Thathandlung" [fact-act], which can only be realised practically. Hegel hence speaks of process and the movement of recognition (Hegel 1971, §430), developing in this context, over several acts, the much-cited master-bondsman scenario (Hegel 1977). The dynamics of these processes are fundamentally incapable of being fully concluded. Being recognised, as the result of the striving for recognition, may be attained eventually within a life story in the framework of fame, esteem, status and so on. However, the development of the I is not thereby automatically concluded, but remains a fragile process, in which attainments can be lost and regained time and again.

As soon as and so long as the *recognition* of the other is related as a result to what is achieved and socially represented, it is ascribable to instrumental seeing. However, in the case of a non-predicating *recognising* of an alterity that cannot be subsumed under identity logic, this inconclusive process character is its crucial ethical quality.[18] Self-consciousness develops, as G. Gamm writes, "through intersubjective processes of mutual acknowledgement. […] In interaction with others, not like a plant, the seed of which already contains all information relevant to its growth" (Gamm 2007).

4 Context and Situation

Reference has already been made several times to one of the essential structural elements of practice: the relation to, and embedding in, given contexts and situations. Activities are generally anchored in cultural and historical contexts and derive their specific sense from each particular situation. This applies to human existence in general[19] as well as to particular cases of human action and speech.[20] Austin and Searle oppose the analysis of language out of context, demonstrating the extent to which the meaning

[18] On the distinction between recognition [Anerkennung] and recognising [Anerkennen], see G. Gamm (2000).

[19] See Nicolai Hartmann (2002), who describes life as "a running chain of coming and going situations".

[20] For Stuart Hampshire (1982), acts are always already situated by virtue of the fact that the human being is at once "observer, actor and language-user."

of a sentence is dependent on its execution in situations. The regulatory context of practice is its involvement in practical contexts that provide its structural preconditions. Whether the sentence 'Sam is coming tomorrow' is a promise or a threat cannot be derived from the sentence itself, since it depends on background phenomena and the situation in which it is pronounced.

The case of seeing is similar. Whether 'Sam sees a piano' means 'he regards himself as prompted to play' or 'he sees an object to which he is entirely indifferent' is contingent on numerous factors. It is, however, never an entirely neutral, receptive procedure without any kind of frame. Hence every perception is a contextually efficient, situated activity.

Whereas context is a term in linguistics and social science, situation is a term that made waves in existentialist philosophy. According to Karl Jaspers, I am only in the world insofar as I am in a situation that defines my "undetermined possibility" (Jaspers 1948, p. 3). I cannot avoid "being in a situation." The term designates a "sense-related reality" (ibid., p. 468f.) that comes from the past, has a history and a future (as possibility and as inevitability), is never entirely finished and permanently changes. Situations demarcate an existential horizon of indetermination, since I find my possibilities constrained within their limits without ever being able to know these limits absolutely.

Both the context and the situation of an epoch and a society condition what is perceivable and how. By taking account of such horizon conditions, it becomes possible to explain the basic duplicity of seeing as responsive and constructive. Situations require that we actively adopt positions and demand decisions that are at the same time reactive and never completely free from external conditions. As Dewey has shown (Dewey 1990, p. 178f.), a situation is not merely the limiting or enabling framework in which I more or less unequivocally realise my pre-set intentions by taking conditions into consideration and deploying the means that the situation puts at my disposal. Rather, the situation functions as a set of conditions in which actors and acts interact such that their mutual dependency softens, if not dissolves the distinction between subject and object.

4.1 Neither Free Nor Arbitrary

Yet it is not only existentially significant situations that condition perceptual practice. Casual and incidental factors and temporal contexts also make contributions. The dependence of perception on context is discussed by

Merleau-Ponty using the example of a film scene by the Russian director Pudovkin involving a close-up of the actor Mozzhukhin with a single facial expression in three different juxtapositions. The first shot follows the image of a bowl of soup, the second that of a dead youth in a coffin and the third that of a child at play. The perception turns the ad hoc into a propter hoc: "The first thing noticed was that Mozzhukhin seemed to be looking at the bowl, the young woman, and the child, and next one noted that he was looking pensively at the dish, that he wore an expression of sorrow when looking at the woman, and that he had a glowing smile for the child. The audience was amazed at his variety of expression although the same shot had actually been used all three times and was, if anything, remarkably inexpressive."[21] The example used by Merleau-Ponty to explain the temporal extension and embeddedness of single acts of perception in a coherent whole shows the influence that the contexts exercise on seeing. Like practice and speech, seeing always takes place in a situation that restricts and binds the viewer and the visible and is specifiable by context-dependent determinations of usage and function. The individual sees and overlooks according to situational and individual dispositions constituted by previous knowledge, propositional approach, evaluative postures and normative assumptions. Beyond this, there are super-individual influences from the given age and culture. People see different things in different ages in different cultures. Landscape, for example, was presumably first seen aesthetically when Petrarca climbed Mont Ventoux. It first became a worthy subject for painting with the Dutch masters of the seventeenth century.

Due to such cultural conditions, which are at once general and particular, individual perception is neither entirely free nor entirely determined. Instead, it is embedded in an intersubjective practice in which historically and socially situated, corporeal individuals act, speak and perceive interdependently. This practice represents the totality of norms, discourses, mores, agreements, power relations and interest within a language and living community.

[21] M. Merleau-Ponty (1964): In film theory, this experiment is attributed to the Soviet director and theorist Lev Kulechov and discussed as the Kulechov effect. See D. Liebsch (2005, p. 77).

5 Form of Life and World Image

Self-purposive seeing at least has a status proximate to that of play, because it is also realised in its performance. Instrumental seeing, on the other hand, is so deeply involved in coping with practical demands that it cannot be described with the notion of play. In the degree to which it serves coping with life, it cannot be either carried out or not carried out voluntarily like play. We cannot choose to participate in it or not. Nor can it be simply replaced by another activity. In order to replace the sense of sight in negotiating the everyday, the blind need to resort to guide dogs, brail, developing the sense of touch and so on.[22]

Yet such comparisons and family resemblances bring us close to the way the practice of seeing is embedded in other performances of living. Many types of seeing have, in common with activities like travelling, reading, sport and playing the flute, the features of self-fulfilling acts—that is, they have an Ενργεια-form characterised by temporal extension and transitory alterability.

Wittgenstein elucidates his theory of meaning as use with the help of the terms 'language game' and 'life form.' Language games clarify how speech and speech acts constitute part of the form of life of a language community. "Here the term 'language-game' is meant to emphasise the fact that the speaking of language is part of an activity, or of a form of life" (Wittgenstein 1986, Part 1, sentence 23). This means that the meaning of signs is not given previously to or outside of their use, but only within a practice and in accordance with this practice. All attempts to explicate the meaning of a word arrive legitimately at their end in language games. Words or sentences have meaning thanks to their embeddedness in social contexts, in language games and forms of life.[23]

The same applies, as I am attempting to demonstrate, for visual activities. Here too, customs and institutions regulate what and how we are capable of seeing and permitted to see. Conventions of seeing do not have the same status as fixed terms within a discursive language game, but they too follow trained interpretive schemata and are prefigured by what Wittgenstein calls

[22]This has been made acutely tangible in the worldwide exhibition 'Dialogue in the Dark,' in which museum visitors are taken through absolutely dark rooms by a blind guide and learn to depend on their hearing, touch, and sense of space.

[23]Controversial commentaries on this term are found in W. Lütterfels (1999) Further: D. Sturma (2001).

a form of life: "What has to be accepted, the given, is—so one could say—forms of life" (Wittgenstein 1986, p. Ilxi). "And to imagine a language means to imagine a form of life" (Wittgenstein 1986, Part 1, Sentence 19). Language, culture and society dictate what can be regarded as agreed and certain, "beyond being justified or unjustified" (Wittgenstein 1969, §359).

The totality of valid norms and ruling convictions, morals, common usage, values and demands, which inform a community's practice, constitute its form of life. Like context but on a more general and thus intangible level, form of life is a rule-giving precondition for possible ways of thinking and perceiving a society and époque: "[human beings] agree in the language they use. That is not agreement in opinions but in form of life" (Wittgenstein 1986, Part 1, Sentence 241).

5.1 Conditions of Possibility and Framing Factors

The problem here, however, is that forms of life are concurrent to all practice, speech and perception, but lie below the threshold of articulation—that is, they are neither discursively explicit nor explicable. This extensional indeterminacy attaches to the term as its systematic characteristic. The form of life works by conditioning like a lens, which we see *through* without being able to see it. We are presumably only capable of understanding why someone sees the way they see on the basis of collective forms of life.

This is also the case for what Wittgenstein refers to as an image of the world or worldview [*Weltbild*]. It is the silent, unexpressed horizon that is not itself discursively explicit, but accompanies everything that is. The Weltbild has worked its way into German speech as the "unquestioned, shared background assumptions that entrench collective reality" (Gamm 1994, p. 132). As the "system of what is believed" (Wittgenstein 1969, §144), "which the speakers of a language regard as the absolutely unquestionable and share among each-other as supra-subjectively valid 'fundamental attitudes'" (Majetschak 2000, p. 355, see Wittgenstein 1969 §238), it conditions what can be said and done and how, without the need for justification.

In my opinion, nothing suggests that the influence of the world image is restricted to language and speaking. It would be inexplicable as to how world images could condition language use while exercising no influence on what can become visible and be seen and in which way.[24]

For this reason, the problems associated with the indeterminacy of these terms are not merely epistemological. More important for our context is the insight that the customs of perception conditioned by images of world and conserved in forms of life reveal and conceal fundamentally and supra-individually the relation between the viewer and the visible. This means that neither the aesthetic freedoms nor moral responsibilities of perceptual world disclosure are merely subjectively constructed; they are instead conditioned by framing principles.

A parallel notion could be elaborated upon by drawing on Husserl's definition of the horizon. As illuminated by G. Gamm, Wittgenstein's concept of the world image fulfils a function similar to Husserl's concept of horizon. "As the incremental horizon or the referential context of appresentation first brings the object out or the determined indeterminacy of the 'pre-'or 'super'-attitude opens the view onto the matter, so too does the worldview first open the possibility of voicing doubt and identifying errors" (Gamm 1994, p. 134).

Yet horizon and world image not only affect possible *beliefs*, they also inform *habits of perception*, influencing what our conventions of seeing make at all perceivable. The horizon and the image affect what is disposed to draw our attention and what can be seen. Just as forms of life regulate, enable and limit language use, while being themselves conceptually ungraspable, invisible horizon factors regulate our interactions with the visible.

Sartre's gaze through the keyhole becomes misconduct only by virtue of the normative horizon of what is the right thing to do, as formulated in images of the world. This context determines, as in speech and practice, which looks are inappropriate, threatening or promising.

6 Acts and Actors

For these reasons it can only be ascertained in particular cases whether a viewer is fascinated, affected, held captive by the visible or, inversely, to what extent she takes hold of the visible, classifies it or keeps it at a distance. Whichever way it is turned, no theory of seeing can do without

[24] On the relation of conditioning between the linguistic and non-linguistic in the context of practice, see Joachim Schulte (1999).

the bipolarity of the viewer and the visible. The decisive thing, however, is to avoid construing the two poles as object-like entities and then leaving it at that, but to locate instead the movement of seeing within their oscillation and interpenetration.

Like practice in general, the act of seeing can be distinguished from experience as a matter of principle in that it is not a pure event of consciousness but rather has a side that is turned to the world or in that it becomes concrete. In individual cases, however, the quality of experience can dominate. Since failing to act is also a type of action, overlooking and selective omission will also have to be understood as activities. These can be active or reactive depending on whether they derive from affective dispositions of the viewer or are due pragmatically to the pressure of a social situation.

Actors are traditionally thought of as more or less autonomous subjects, acting with reasons from a particular starting position and oriented toward certain ends. There are, however, many debates over whether or not the term action necessarily requires such an intentional actor sure of her aims. More recent theories of practice have distanced themselves from this conception, understanding practice rather as an interaction between acts and actors, structures and concerns. Pragmatic theories of practice emphasise that human action does not spring from an isolated, deliberately planned act but is rather part of definite social practices and explicable out of the situational texture of closely woven actions in whose performance the actors are co-operators in a world of things that they at once express, use and suffer. The non-explicit, collective criteria of practice, the normative preconditions and criteria of judgement are due not to individual convictions alone but are rather constituted out of practical social interconnections. Any notion that separates and reifies the individual elements of practice necessarily obscures their interaction and temporal continuity.

The agent of the event of vision can certainly not be grasped by the scheme from classical practice theory. The concept of an active subject as a voluntary and sapient actor making decisions and realising goals is too gross to illuminate the variously conditioned character of intersubjective practice. The viewer must be described differently. A weaker concept of the actor as retroactive and responding to demands, interests and appeals is presumably more appropriate for describing the seeing subject, who always sees from their own individual perspective but at the same time always has to react in some way or other to something visible. It would seem to be crucial to avoid considering the viewer as someone engaged in a separate activity. From Merleau-Ponty to Goodman, it has repeatedly been pointed out that the viewer perceives with her whole self, her corporeality and her socialisation. Although she cannot plan what she sees, she will still see what she expects to see. She has *learnt* to see. This fact is also relevant to understanding the social and historical conditioning of perception. She has developed perceptual customs based on culture, gender and personality. She sees according to both 'private' and 'public' preconditions.

7 Medium and Mediality

The distinction between medium and mediality can be put to work in the same way as that between the instrumental and the self-purposive, between means and ends. Seeing as a purpose-serving means to an end implies the use of the eyes as an object-like tool such as a telescope or a magnifying glass—classical instruments for mediating perception.[25] It is entirely different to be seeing in those cases where we see ourselves and are ourselves visible as we move about in the world, looking involuntarily and non-intentionally. Perception is then more like the element we find ourselves in than a medium of which we make use. As medial occurrence, seeing is a way of relating to something that at the same time absorbs us.

There is again a striking similarity to the way language is constituted. Where language is something we move about in and at the same time the means by which we communicate, so too is perception characterised by a thoroughly paradox duplicity. Neither the world nor the other are immediately given but rather mediated and generated by language and perception.

The tension between the concept of mediality and that of action is, in my opinion, resolved in the concept of practice, since it already entails the various component parts—that is, the purpose-serving and the executive, or, in other words, the determinable and the determined. The concept of action requires an actor, whereas mediality instead expresses the character of something happening. Now, seeing always entails something of both. It can be both functional and directed at ends and also casual and involuntary. It can focus on something or be captured by something. Practice is itself the umbrella term for these logical paradoxes. In practice, the medial character of seeing can interact with its character as action. The odd medial

[25] Interesting material on this topic can be found in the anthology from E. Fischer-Lichte (2001).

location of practice between subject and object is precisely its specific feature. Furthermore, since the actors in perceptual practice are usually not autonomous active subjects carrying out plans, there is no real contradiction in it being simultaneously an activity and a happening. Mediality enters into play where intentional, seeking or predicating seeing is replaced by seeing as an encounter or exchange—that is, the exchange between the visible and the viewer. As we have seen, the logic of the exchange is also a constitutive element of practice.

Because seeing is always a movement between two poles, between consciousness and world, the sensory and the mental, reception and spontaneity, it must itself be a mediating movement. It always proceeds as a balancing act that can lean toward at least two different sides, or rather originates from two different sources. Such a mediating activity cannot be thought of as a relation between objects in which someone gives something to someone else, like a real estate agent finding someone a house. In such a relation, the medium and the thing being mediated are each already there as objects and can be easily distinguished. The paradox of perceptual practice is that the physical world as such is not an object, but rather the result of a process conditioned by individual and socio-cultural criteria. The strange thing here is that something is at the same time found and invented.

7.1 Mediated Immediacy

The mediality of seeing can perhaps be described with Helmuth Plessner's concept of mediated immediacy. Plessner's concept seems capable of terminologically grasping a relation that cannot be described as either subjective or objective. The whole of human existence in its duplicity of *being* a body and *having* a body involves the simultaneity of immediate affectivity and mediated reflective distance. Plessner refers to this as eccentric positionality: "Eccentricity of position can be understood as a position in which the living subject is in indirect-direct relation to everything. Indirect-direct relation should be understood as the form of connection in which the connecting joint is necessary to produce the immediacy of the connection" (Plessner 1975, p. 324). In these sentences, we find the attempt to avoid a discrete subject-object-onotology by replacing it with a set of mutual conditions whose components cannot be thought of independently of one another. Relocated to the context being dealt with here, the paradox figure of mediated immediacy can be applied to the relation of mutual determination embracing the viewer and the visible. Perceptual world disclosure is both a mediated and immediate form of relation to self and world, because in perception something is at once constituted and pre-existent; something sensory is produced such that response and spontaneity interact.

The concept of practice provides an alternative to the subject-object-scheme by clearly showing the way both are mediated by their situation in contexts and forms of life. Practice means being visible to oneself and to others, acting and speaking in the world as a place we inhabit collectively, not infrequently fighting about its sense as a whole. We have incidentally seen that seeing can largely be divided into a functional-pragmatic and a self-purposive dimension, whereby the many and varied applications of visual perception can be systematically classified.

References

Adorno, Theodor W. 1977. Kulturkritik. In *Gesammelte Schriften*, Vol. 10, 2. Frankfurt am Main: Suhrkamp.

Arendt, Hannah. 1958. *The Human Condition*. Chicago: University of Chicago Press.

Aristotle. 2000. *Nicomachean Ethics*. Cambridge: Cambridge University Press.

Austin, John Langshaw. 1961. *Philosophical Papers*. Oxford: Oxford University Press.

Austin, John Langshaw. 1975. *How to Do Things with Words*. Cambridge: Harvard University Press.

Böhme, Gernot. 2000. *Theorie des Bildes*. Munich: Fink.

Bourdieu, Pierre. 1990. *The Logic of Practice*. Stanford: Stanford University Press.

Bourdieu, Pierre. 1991. *Language and Symbolic Power*. Cambridge: Polity Press.

Bourdieu, Pierre. 1998. *Theory of Action*. Stanford: Stanford University Press.

Bubner, Rüdiger. 1976. *Handlung, Sprache und Vernunft. Grundbegriffe praktischer Philosophie*. Frankfurt am Main: Suhrkamp.

Butler, Judith. 1997. *The Psychic Life of Power: Theories in Subjection*. Stanford: Stanford University Press.

Crutchfield, Richard S. (ed.). 1982. *Elements of Psychology*. New York: A. Knopf.

Dewey, John. 1990. *The Later Works: 1925–1953, Vol. 4: 1929: The Quest for Certainty*. Carbondale: Southern Illinois University Press.

Ducasse, Curt John. 1951. *Nature, Mind and Death*. La Salle: The Open Court Publishing Company.

Düsing, Edith. 1986. *Intersubjektivität und Selbstbewußtsein*. Köln: Dinter.

Fichte, Johann Gottlieb. 2000. *Foundations of Natural Right*. Cambridge: Cambridge University Press.

Fischer-Lichte, Erika, et al. (eds.). 2001. *Wahrnehmung und Medialität*. Tübingen: Francke.

Gamm, Gerhard. 1994. *Flucht aus der Kategorie*. Frankfurt am Main: Suhrkamp.
Gamm, Gerhard. 2000. *Nicht Nichts*, 213–224. Frankfurt am Main: Suhrkamp.
Gamm, Gerhard. 2007. Stehen. In *Wörterbuch philosophischer Metaphern*, ed. Ralf Konersmann, 420–432. Darmstadt: Wissenschaftliche Buchgesellschaft.
Gehlen, Arnold. 1966. *Der Mensch*, 157–180. Frankfurt am Main: Athenäum.
Goldstein, E. Bruce. 2002. *Sensation and Perception*. Pacific Grove: Wadsworth.
Hampshire, Stuart. 1982. Persons and Their Situations. In *Thought and Action*, 11–89. London: Chatto and Windus.
Hartmann, Nicolai. 2002. *Moral Phenomena: Volume One of Ethics*. New Brunswick: Transaction Publishers.
Hartmut, Böhme. 2004. Das Unsichtbare. In *Performativität und Medialität*, ed. Sybille Krämer, 215–246. Munich: Fink.
Hegel, Georg Wilhelm Friedrich. 1971. *Encyclopaedia of Philosophical Sciences*. Oxford: Clarendon.
Hegel, Georg Wilhelm Friedrich. 1977. *Phenomenology of Spirit*. Oxford: Oxford University Press.
Hegemann, Carl Georg. 1982. *Identität und Selbst-Zerstörung*. Frankfurt am Main: Campus-Verlag.
Heidegger, Martin. 1962. *Kant and the Problem of Metaphysics*. Bloomington: Indiana University Press.
Honneth, Axel. 1996. *The Struggle for Recognition: The Moral Grammar of Social Conflicts*. Cambridge: The MIT Press.
Honneth, Axel. 2003. *Unsichtbarkeit*. Frankfurt am Main: Suhrkamp.
Humboldt, Wilhelm von. 1973. *Schriften zur Sprache*. Stuttgart: Reclam.
Husserl, Edmund. 1997. *Thing and Space*. Dordrecht: Springer.
Husserl, Edmund. 1999. *Cartesian Meditations*. Dordrecht: Kluwer.
Jaspers, Karl. 1948. *Philosophie*. Berlin: Springer.
Kant, Immanuel. 1998. *Critique of Pure Reason*. London and Cambridge: Cambridge University Press.
Kobbert, Max Jürgen. 1982. *Kunstpsychologie: Kunstwerk, Künstler und Betrachter*. Darmstadt: WBG.
Lévinas, Emmanuel. 1969. *Totality and Infinity*. Pittsburgh: Duquesne University Press.
Liebsch, Dimitri (ed.). 2005. *Philosophie des Films*. Paderborn: Mentis.
Lütterfels, Wilhelm, et al. (ed.). 1999. *Der Konflikt der Lebensformen in Wittgensteins Philosophie der Sprache*. Frankfurt am Main: Suhrkamp.
Majetschak, Stefan. 2000. *Ludwig Wittgensteins Denkweg*. Munich: Alber.
Mead, George Hebert. 1912. The Mechanism of Social Consciousness. *Journal of Philosophy, Psychology and Scientific Methods* 9 (15): 401–406.
Mead, George Herbert. 1992. *Mind, Self, and Society: From the Standpoint of a Social Behaviorist*. Chicago: University of Chicago Press.

Merleau-Ponty, Maurice. 1964. The Film and the New Psychology. In *Sense and Non-Sense*, 48–59. Evanston: Northwestern University Press.
Merleau-Ponty, Maurice. 1973. *Adventures of the Dialectic*. Evanston: Northwestern University Press.
Merleau-Ponty, Maurice. 2004. *Basic Writings*. London: Routledge.
Morris, Charles William. 1970. *Foundations of the Theory of Signs*. Chicago: University of Chicago Press.
Plessner, Helmuth. 1975. *Die Stufen des Organischen und der Mensch*. Berlin: de Gruyter.
Proust, Marcel. 1993. In *Search of Lost Time, Vol. VI: Time Regained*. New York: Modern Library.
Sartre, Jean-Paul. 1992. *Being and Nothingness*. New York: Washington Square Press.
Schulte, Joachim. 1999. Die Hinnahme von Sprachspielen und Lebensformen. In *Der Konflikt der Lebensformen in Wittgensteins Philosophie der Sprache*, ed. Wilhelm Lütterfels et al., 156–170. Frankfurt am Main: Suhrkamp.
Searle, John Rogers. 1969. *Speech Acts*. Cambridge: Cambridge University Press.
Seel, Martin. 2002. *Sich bestimmen lassen. Studien zur theortischen und praktischen Philosophie*, 278–298. Frankfurt am Main: Suhrkamp.
Siep, Ludwig. 1979. *Anerkennung als Prinzip der praktischen Philosophie*. Munich: Alber.
Strawson, Peter Frederick. 1964. Intention and Convention in Speech Acts. *The Philosophical Review* 73 (4): 439–460.
Sturma, Dieter. 2001. Philosophie und Lebensform. In *Anerkennung*, ed. Monika Hofmann-Riedinger et al., 170–183. Freiburg: Alber.
Wertheimer, Max. 1974. The Problem of Perceptual Structure. In *Handbook of Perception*, Vol 1, 75–91, ed. Edward C. Carterette et al. New York: Academic Press.
Wiesing, Lambert (ed.). 2002. *Philosophie der Wahrnehmung*. Suhrkamp: Frankfurt am Main.
Wildt, Andreas. 1982. *Autonomie und Anerkennung*. Stuttgart: Klett-Cotta.
Wittgenstein, Ludwig. 1969. *On Certainty*. Oxford: Blackwell.
Wittgenstein, Ludwig. 1986. *Philosophical Investigations*. Oxford: Basil Blackwell.

CHAPTER 4

The Performativity of Practice

You have to make something new in order to see something new.[1]

A concept of practice that breaks with the traditional distinction between subject and object cannot dispose of the individual agent. All seeing presupposes someone doing the seeing, even though the existence of this person does not explain entirely what seeing is. In the interplay with other agents of the perceptual practice, viewers are executors of a performative event that itself brings about what the practice determines and enables. Practice involves not only the potential and the actual in a relation of mutual determination, it also implies a dimension of individuality. Yet there is no reason to suppose that this individuality is a freely constructed subjectivity or that the visible world is discretely objective. Rather, the practical is a non-reified process of exchange between the viewer and the visible—a mediating movement between self and world. Practice, in the sense of the non-reified process involving a relation of mutual determination encompassing actors, acts and contexts can only occur at all by being *done*. This notion will help demonstrate the interpretive, selective and variable character of seeing as a perceptual practice.

[1] G. C. Lichtenberg (1984, J 1310).

E. Schuermann, *Seeing as Practice*, Performance Philosophy,
https://doi.org/10.1007/978-3-030-14507-1_4

Considering that seeing is a constitutive act, how can its reactive and receptive character as an encounter with something be explained? Methodically formulated, the problem is to conceptualise seeing in such a way as to avoid the one-sided approach of both phenomenological essentialism and constructivist relativism. This can perhaps only be attained with concepts themselves duplicitous in their logical constitution.

The power of the performance model depends not only on its place in the philosophy of language but also on its role in the theory of presentation.[2] As Christiaan Hart Nibbrig suggests, presentation is the "performative act that produces something of a sort that didn't previously exist" (Hart Nibbrig 1994). I want to add to this the consideration that the performance of a perception can be seen to resemble formulation in speech in being an act of articulation, a non-reified presentation of the thing seen. Someone sees something that shows itself to her, such that the mode—the *how*—determines the *what*.

The performativity of such seeing could be referred to as a medial event or process. As S. Krämer has explained, the terms performativity and mediality "mediate something and in so doing generate it" (Krämer 2004, p. 23). As has been shown in the chapter on practice, the mediality of perception resides in its participation in any active relation between self and world. This simultaneity of mediation and generation is fundamental for a theory of seeing. Such concepts can describe the interplay between the receptive and generative properties of seeing. The terms help to describe how seeing can be an encounter with the visible world—in the sense of a quiddity—and at the same time a production of that world by determining *how* it is perceived. Thus, the way visible things address us can be mediated with the aspect-character of seeing. Both mediative and generative dimensions of seeing are constituents of practice.

1 Doing as Depicting

The performance of seeing can be differentiated into an instrumental and a self-purposive dimension. If looking can produce illocutionary effects such as warning or promising, then the practice of perception is analogous to Austinian performatives, as explained above. However, when I look about

[2] An introduction to the breadth of use of the term is provided by the anthologies U. Wirth (2002), J. Kertscher and D. Mersch (2003), further: C. Wulf and J. Zirfas (2005).

distractedly or am submersed in the contemplation of a painting, the performativity of the event resides in a less goal-oriented type of seeing with no tangible result. Just as I can walk for pleasure, or alternatively with the express purpose of reaching a specific destination, so too can seeing be either disinterested or directed towards an end. Yet it always remains performance, always 'at work.' The performativity of seeing is its individual form of execution.

As Austin's version of speech act theory has shown, speech cannot be reduced to the instrumental use of language and the predicative semantics of propositional content. Speech cannot simply be explained without considering the way it is performed. The meaning of the activity of speech is not primarily to be understood from the proposition, but rather from the execution character of the real act. With attention to the performativity of speech, the act of speaking becomes more significant than the thing spoken; the speaker's voice, cadence, flow, volume and accompanying elements of expression such as a quivering of the voice or a sharpness of tone come into view. Briefly put, the result of the speech act is considered here on its own terms, independently of propositional content.

A theory of seeing can borrow from this approach. Visual perception is not conceivable outside of a particular execution; it is realised in the course of being performed. Seeing cannot be reduced to the thing seen any more than speech to the thing spoken. However, this analogy reaches its limit in cases where the perlocutionary effects of seeing are not as tangible as in communicative seeing, because it is instead the *how* of execution that decides *what* something is seen *as*. This *how* is better described with the notion of performativity drawn from the theory of representation. In the way a pictorial or theatrical representation shows the thing presented in a particular light, in a particular way, seeing also 'shows' the seen as something that is never quite neutral, as it is always perceived from a particular angle under a particular aspect. Showing and seeing are showing *as* and seeing *as* in that they are always aspect-like.

Although the presentational form of seeing lacks manifest objectification, it precedes the totality of objectifications, remaining inherent to each. The way the director sees is inherent to the film, the way the painter sees is inherent to the picture. Seeing the world with a particular *way of seeing* precedes the way this seeing is expressed in language. The phrasing is chosen according to the mode of seeing. In the performance of seeing, process and result coincide.

Before turning to the presentational potency and semantic capacity to produce sense in the performance of seeing, the structural elements of the performative act of perception need to be more clearly elucidated.

1.1 Space, Time and Perspective

The performativity of the act of seeing can be clearly seen in its spatio-temporal extension and perspectival constitution. Because it is performance, seeing cannot be a conclusive act, but is rather a continuously changing progression. With their stereoscopic ability to see depth, the eyes move about in a visible world also in motion, with both the eyes and world constantly in the flux of generation and transformation. The mobility of the eyes is the enabling condition of the possibility of seeing motion, as well as for seeing objects, which vary according to changes in light.

Seeing is perspectival because all performative self and world relations must presuppose a point of view (standpoint and directedness). As Nietzsche showed, there would be no world without perspectives. Every act of seeing can therefore only realise aspects of possible visibility. If every act of seeing is not aspect-seeing in the Wittgensteinian sense, it is because seeing something is not the same as seeing something *as something*. Yet seeing something is also constrained by perspective. The Necker cube that can only be seen from a certain perspective illustrates this phenomenon: "C'est le point de vue qui crée l'objet" [The object is created by the point of view] (de Saussure 1976, p. 22).

From a particular starting point, seeing traverses spaces and in-between spaces, it *engages* and *starts up*, it creates continuities and breaks, sees forwards and backwards. The ability to distinguish near and far in perception invests the visual world with body and depth. Binocular seeing combines the views of an object from the different locations of the eyes into a spatial unity.

The temporal dimension of both vision and the visible imparts a fading quality to perceptions; they do not manifest as a final, external form but rather constantly advance and recede in transition from self to other, as transformation, modulation or as a movement without a telos.

The executive character of seeing is constituted both inchoately as the introduction of something novel and in pre-emption of something we are expecting, as well as in reconstructing something already seen. Seeing is always 'here and now,' hic et nunc. It is simultaneous in this respect, even when it wanders about successively in space in order to gradually attain certainty. As attention to the present, it is always 'now'. The untranslatable German word *Augenblick* [literally 'glimpse of an eye,' meaning moment, instant] expresses the simultaneity of the temporal and the visual. The optical and the temporal of the Augenblick converge in the look [*Blick*], in the *now* of the presence of looking and being looked at.

At the same time, seeing is given temporal extension by reaching for things invisible, things absent to the senses, by memories that complete the vision and by prefiguring expectations. What Bergson asserts about listening to music (Bergson 2004) also applies to seeing. The power of memory and its influence on expectation within perception extends over a stretch of time, creating cohesive duration. Like the light of a burnt-out star, a past perception comes late to consciousness and re-colours the perception of the present. The process character manifests not only in the floating gaze but also when attention is redirected by other mental processes like wishing or believing. Things not present to vision that would have to be viewed from another angle are revealed gradually. Or there are suddenly emerging, new perspectives causing something to appear in a different light, such that something old and familiar can be seen in a new way. Certainly, this does not only apply to perception, since other events and experiences might be required additionally. However, to the extent that seeing and ways of seeing are interconnected, seeing the novel and seeing differently are dependent on forms of aisthetic performance.

The distinction in English between gaze and glance,[3] focussed look and fleeting look, applied by N. Bryson to viewing painting, also applies outside of aesthetics. The gaze is an arresting, freezing [*festschreiben*; literally to fix in writing] seeing that puts things in static pigeonholes. Glance, on the other hand, is a roving look [*schweifender Blick*], as transient as the passing moment [*Augenblick*], which takes up the apparition in its own temporality. This distinction is illuminating despite Bryson's critique of ideology, which reserves the gaze more or less for the Western, disciplined logic of the look, while grasping the glance as paradigmatic for the Eastern type of seeing. The terminological distinction remains relevant to the temporal factor of seeing regardless of how this is decided. The determining gaze corresponds to the type of seeing described here as instrumental and useful, while the glance exhibits the character of self-purposive performance.

[3]N. Bryson (1983). With this distinction, Norman Bryson attempts to overcome Gombrich's psychology of perception and show how Western Art is socially and historically determined.

1.2 *The Corporeality and Affectivity of Seeing*

Perception is unthinkable without the 'as-structure' of consciousness we discussed earlier. Yet the person seeing does not act as a world-less, rational subject, but rather in a collectively negotiated world of interdependent activity, speech and perception, in which she perceives with her entire person—that ism, with the series of "epistemic and moral attitudes" (Sturma 2005, p. 243)[4] that constitute personhood. The personal attitudes and presumptions Bourdieu refers to as habitus prefigure attention. The agents of seeing are, so to speak, tied up; they are responsively and interactively anchored in what they perceive. In the aisthetic, the simultaneity of determining and being determined that constitutes practice means that the agents are affected to at least the same extent as they actively engage in identifying something. In the situational interweaving of closely bound up practices, such agents are co-agents.

Many authors, from James Gibson (Gibson 1966) to Hermann Schmitz (Schmitz 1967) and Maurice Merleau-Ponty, have stressed that seeing is based on bodily familiarity with the world as a pre-theoretical, meaningful context. Gibson referred to this as "keeping-in-touch with the world" (Gibson 1986, p. 239). Merleau-Ponty understands it as being touched by and touching the world in which our self is rooted. Thus anchored in embodiment, perception is at once active and passive: "my gaze pairs off with colour, and my hand with hardness and softness, and in this transaction between the subject of sensation and the sensible it cannot be held that one acts while the other suffers the action" (Merleau-Ponty 1962, p. 214). The body is not merely one object among many; it is itself the condition for anything to become an object—always there, accompanying everything. For this reason, Merleau-Ponty rejects the notion that the look can determine the way it wanders about among things. Rather, it finds itself together with things inside a shared horizon, the structure of simultaneous possibility and impossibility that prefigures the perceptible. For everything perceptible to the body it holds true that "I perceive in a total way with my whole being; I grasp a unique structure of the thing, a unique way of being, which speaks to all my senses at once" (Merleau-Ponty 1964, p. 49).

Affective dispositions are also closely bound up with the corporeality of the visual process. Wishes and fears will be dealt with further on in connection with the imagination. There we will see that imagination often

[4] For a more detailed account of the concept of personhood (Sturma 1997).

contributes to motivating interpersonal seeing. Because of its reciprocity, this type of seeing is least capable of being 'neutral' and disengaged.

Studies in the psychology of perception also show that needs such as hunger alter the focus of perception; for example, when incomplete words are completed to make them denote food (Crutchfield 1982). The willingness to perceive what we want increases to the point where we think we see what we need. Gibson rightly spoke of seeing as a 'psychosomatic act' (Gibson 1986, p. 240). Someone who is disgusted by the sight of spiders or raw meat is not fabricating constructs that she can pick and choose at will. She is instead determined by perceptions forced upon her by her physical being-in-the-world.

A first-person perspective, non-sharable with others, and qualitative perceptions are the conditions of the body. The body also constitutes a relation to self, referred to by Plessner as ex-centricity. The duplicity of *being* a body and *having* a body is responsible for an ex-centric relation to self, involving difference. This difference reoccurs at the level of perception to the extent that the viewer in her corporeality is herself a visible object among others. The corporeality of the viewer is conditioned by what she perceives with her total, corporeal being-in-the-world,[5] and this corporeality is the condition for her visibility to others.

The performative dimension of seeing, the way seeing embodies expression, is particularly conspicuous in the act of seeing persons, since being physically visible to the other is always, in some way, socially meaningful. Performative processes are embodiments; they transpose something into a three- dimensional act. The visible body is a means of expression and is itself the process by which social reality is brought about. As Judith Butler explains, "The 'I' that is its body is, of necessity, a mode of embodying, and the 'what' that it embodies is possibilities" (Butler 1988, p. 521). "[T]he possibilities that are embodied are not fundamentally exterior or antecedent to the process of embodying itself" (ibid.). And yet they must be analytically distinguishable from each other. The body is thus a socio-historical situation as well as the continuous reproduction of that situation.

[5] The integration of the body in seeing and the usefulness of seeing as an alternative form of touch is illustrated by Volkmar Mühleis'(2005) study of work by artists limiting the dominance of the visual in visual arts by dealing with haptic and holistic types of experience.

1.3 Negativity and Blindness

To claim that seeing is performance is also to take into account the negative side of the process. Seeing something entails blocking out or overlooking other things. A figure can only be focussed upon by making the background vanish. The periphery of view is populated by colours and forms that we only partially perceive. Vagueness is a necessary element of any exercise of vision. Partial and casual seeing are integral parts of the visible world of which only a slice is ever realised, while the greater part remains invisible. We have already mentioned types of habitual blindness; no longer seeing familiar things or overlooking things we are accustomed to interpreting schematically. The practice of seeing systematically involves overlooking things, reducing things and blocking things out. This has been aptly described by Gehlen: "First the overlooking of countless possible perceptions provides an overview [...] In this way the world as a field of surprises *reduced* to sequences of 'overlooked' centres" (Gehlen 1966, p. 173f).

The blind spot—in physiological terms, the point of contact between the optic nerve and the retina—corresponds psychologically to the individual's desire not to see something.

The negativity of vision is what makes its essential creativity comprehensible by explaining how our perceptions can diverge from what is given to visibility. What we see and, more importantly, what we do not see result from acts of selection that individualise the meaning of the seen.

Like the negativity of the visible, the negativity of seeing must be subdivided. To overlook something is different from being blinded by imaginings. Supplementary seeing and selective seeing are each woven into the invisible differently. The former not only completes a seen object by adding its other sides, but also adds inventions, interpretations and imaginings. We not only do not see what we do not see, we also do not see *that* we do not see it (Foerster 1985). Moreover, the performance of vision is itself never visible.

Seeing is interspersed with specific blind spots just as the invisible and the visible intertwine mutually. These blind spots are due to the affective and imaginary context in which the process of perception is embedded. Yet the process is selective even without such affective conditioning, since it always involves blindness to specific things. Even a largely constative perception without the participation of imagination has its own characteristic blindness; for example, to the aesthetic attraction of a particular phenomenon or to its social meaning. Interestingly, even the age-old notion of the innocent eye, of a neutral impartial perception, is discredited by the participation of blindness in all seeing. As Tom Mitchell has shown, even if an innocent eye existed, it would in no way 'objectively' see the way things are. "When we try to postulate a foundational experience of 'pure' vision, a merely mechanical process uncontaminated by imagination, purpose, or desire, we invariably discover one of the few maxims on which Gombrich and Nelson Goodman agree: 'the innocent eye is blind.' The capacity for a purely physical vision that is supposed to be forever inaccessible to the blind turns out to be itself a kind of blindness" (Mitchell 1986, p. 118). Even if pure perception were to exist, which both Gombrich and Goodman deny, it would be partially blind to the possible social meanings of the seen.

Operations have been performed on people born blind to make them capable of retinal reactions and thus, in theory, physiologically capable of seeing, but whose brains recognise nothing from visual stimuli, such that they are unable to report what is in front of them. This confirms that seeing is socially learnt and must be informed by imagination. A further phenomenon is that of blind sight, in which cortically blind patients can nevertheless locate stimuli in their field of vision when asked[6] (Goldstein 2002, p. 77f). The patient can receive information, but this information is not suitably processed into conscious experience to permit her to report it. Blind sight patients obviously retain certain previous intact experiences of the visible. In his theory of consciousness, Colin McGinn concludes from this that "there is a component of experience in normal seeing that is not subject to introspection" (McGinn 1999, p. 148). This means that visual perception takes in more than is accessible to consciousness. McGinn continues: "When I see a prickly green cactus in bloom there is more to this experience than is apparent to my introspective eye; it also harbours a hidden set of properties, not given to introspection. Just as there is more to the cactus itself than is evident in my perception of it (its cellular structure, for example), so there is more to my visual experience of the cactus than the way this experience strikes me from the inside" (ibid., p. 148,149). In other words, not everything that occurs in perception is present to consciousness. In blind sight patients, the unconscious part seems to have become autonomous. The part of seeing that becomes conscious would thus always be less than the whole. The difficulty involved in putting colour impressions into words addresses this problem from another side.

[6] For a more detailed account see L. Weiskrantz (1986).

2 The What and the How

The foregoing overview of the performative structural elements of seeing has made it clear that the interrelation of the see-er and the seen, of perception and blindness in their individual spatio-temporal and corporeal situations, implies that ways of seeing hang together not only with conclusions that are distinct or distinguishable from perception, but also that such ways of seeing start out from the act of seeing. The capacity of seeing itself to organise and interpret informs *how* we see something and *what* we can perceive it as. This capacity invests seeing with its *iconicity*, which will concern us in what follows.

The comparison with speaking should again serve to clarify this point. Words and sentences have undertones; they are fortified or countered by gestures. Voice and cadence can be more significant than the content of an utterance. Understanding others does not consist in just hearing their words. Sometimes the voice can betray what the words are trying to conceal. The expressive force of this type of speech is constitutive of the semantic content of the utterance.

The *how* of seeing represents a comparable case. Relations to self and world are articulated not only via speech but also aisthetically. In the practice of seeing, what is perceived is developed into a figure. Seeing can be compared to speech as a form of expression because it also produces and organises sense on its own in sensory receptivity, prior to subsequent acts of judgement. The shaping function of speech that Humboldt refers to as its "Geisteseigentümlichkeit" [idiosyncratic mental characteristic] (Humboldt 1973, p. 32 ff) could correspond to a "Wahrnehmungseigentümlichkeit" [idiosyncratic perceptual characteristic] inherent in all performers of seeing.

Unlike speech, however, these processes of sense production remain immanent to consciousness. They are not expressed in a medium comparable to the voice,[7] nor do they materialise in visible pictures. The reflective translation of perceptions into speech is needed for communication between subjects in which ways of seeing play a part. This does not alter the fact that formative and quasi-representational principles are operative in seeing. Indeed, it is necessary to include imaginative participation in the

[7] Although the voice too is characterised by sonic performance, it is a subjectively perceptible medium of expression. The expressivity of seeing, however, must first be put into speech in order to be perceptible to others. See the anthology D. Kolesch and S. Krämer (2006).

concept of seeing. The practice of seeing involves the constant and constitutive participation of creative imaginings, or, more simply, the faculty of imagination referred to by Kant in the *Critique of the Faculty of Judgement* as the "faculty of representation."[8] (Kant 2000, §§17, 23, 49, 62)

2.1 The Fictional and Narrative Constitution of Reality

There is a further semantic sense in which a comparison between acts of seeing and speech acts is illuminating—namely, in the analogy that seeing is to pictures as speech is to stories. Speech is a way of representing lived experience in narrative. In narration, life solidifies to story. Hannah Arendt shows that stories are indeed the actual products of speech and activity. Life, in its openness to a future, is a story the ending of which is uncertain—except in that it ends fatally. Living human beings can cope with moving toward their own death as the only certain end, without acting as if they were waiting for a death sentence, because they are always already entangled in stories. (Arendt 1959). The meaning of stories is first revealed when life itself has come to an end. The suspense of how life stories are going to turn out generally prevents the owners of the stories from losing their vital spirits. This can only be explained by activity, as Hannah Arendt points out, because this alone is self-purposive performance, the finality of which is uncertain. The act of production looks towards its end as its foreseeable result.

Narrative is therefore represented activity. Actions and experiences are configured together by means of the malleable capacities of storytelling to account for the reasons and motives of action. Narrative has not only an aesthetic status, it serves also to ethically legitimate actions by giving reasons. When someone is asked for reasons for action, she immediately enters a synthetic act of storytelling. Stories introduce perspectives into practice that order or 'falsify' without general criteria for falsehood and truthfulness. MacIntyre's (MacIntyre 2007, p. 206ff.) simple but instructive example of a man working in the garden makes this clear. Whether or not he is doing his wife a favour, preparing for the winter or getting some exercise is a question of point of view. And the point of view depends on which relation

[8] The faculty of Imagination as a form of representation is the main inspiration for Lyotard's reading of Kant. See J.-F. Lyotard (1988).

is assumed to exist between causes or intentions and the activity itself.[9] Stories create meaning by assuming points of view from which to attribute reasons and intentions and determine contexts.

Donald Davidson has advocated understanding reasons for actions as causes, and rationalisations as "causal explanations" (Davidson 2001, p. 4). Reasons based on the beliefs and evaluative attitudes of the actor cause her to act. What role a given motive plays and when, is a question of internal and external interpretation contingent on speech acts. Intentions can only be got at via self-explanations, retrospection and interpretation. From the first-person perspective, intentions are already contingent on rationalisation that can be found after the event and could not have been clear and evident to the actors a priori. From the observer perspective, finally, intentions are broadly intangible and difficult to pronounce upon. In any case, the interpretation of lived experience is not entirely arbitrary but rather an unavoidable condition of life, as life reflecting on itself. Narrative is a representative way to cope with life in ethical and aesthetic terms.

In what follows, I will develop the performance of semantic *seeing something as something* as a mode of fictional, configurating representation, which is comparable to narration in that it is close to explanation and understanding in the way speech is to narration and representation. Interpretations and images issue from seeing with the same sort of logical development as stories follow from speech and activity. The way narration oscillates between discovery and invention manifests structural similarities to the paradoxical duplicity of perception in its oscillation between constitution and response. Perception is extremely difficult to separate out from the insights and knowledge it enables and mediates. If we consider the relation as consisting between occasion and result, we again isolate seeing from judgement. This is dictated by the order of theory but is not true to the way that perception and knowledge are interwoven in practice. It is characteristic of all action in practice that it always bears relations to

[9] Is he doing his wife a favour by getting some exercise or by preparing the garden for winter? Or is doing his wife a favour only incidental to his actual concern of getting some exercise in the fresh air? If he were to keep digging while his beliefs about his wife changed, the framework of the story would also change. In the first instance, it would be the story of a practical measure in a household with garden. In the second instance, a story about a husband's relationship with his wife. The intentions cannot be described independently of the interpretive point of view. They must be divided into primary and secondary status. Activities thus become what they are by contextualisation. See also the discussion of Charles Taylor in Chap. I.2.c.

knowledge, feeling and conviction because it is embedded in the whole of a socially shaped life. This involvement is even more pertinent to the act of seeing, which exhibits both the aspect of consciousness in experience and the aspect of world in activity. In seeing, the world shows itself in different ways that nevertheless do not attain to objective expression. The perceptual images remain constructions inside consciousness.

2.2 Style and (Re)Formulation

Although they are processes of consciousness, *how* I see something and how something presents itself to me exhibit commonalities with objectified pictorial representation. Individual ways of seeing are perceptible in the same way in which style causes an artistic representation—whether linguistic or pictorial—to come into being in an individual way. Just as every human being has a personal style of speaking, the stylistic character of habitual perspectives could be a decisive factor in the practice of seeing.

Marcel Proust may well have been thinking of this when he qualified style as 'vision': "for style for the writer [...] is a question not of technique but of vision: it is the revelation, which by direct and conscious methods would be impossible, of the qualitative difference, the uniqueness of the fashion in which the world appears to each one of us, a difference which, if there were no art, would remain forever the secret of every individual" (Proust 1993, p. 299).

This qualitative difference in the way we see will continue to concern us here. The individual ways painters and writers see is manifested in their work when it becomes visible and interpretable for others. The otherwise invisible execution of an act of seeing is rendered sensibly perceptible in its products, making it an act of expression. Comparable pictorial capacities are presumably at play when non-artists see, though they remain intrinsic, representing a kind of 'je ne sais quoi' of individual perception.

Merleau-Ponty's characterisation of style as "a mode of formulation" (Merleau-Ponty 1993, p. 254) indicates that the way something is expressed is a representative, constitutive act manifesting itself equally on the levels of syntax, semantics and pragmatics.[10] Performative acts of formulation similar to those executed by actors or professional radio announcers when they transform a literary text into a performance, can transform

[10] See for instance M. Frank (1990, p. 11ff.). Also helpful is the article by Rainer Rosenberg (2003).

seeing into an expressive or presentational, constitutional event. The art of the radio play, for example, is largely reliant on the art of the speakers and the presentational quality of their formulations. In contrast to a stage actor who can work with gesture, facial expression and stage presence, the speaker in a radio play relies entirely on voice, tone and speech acts. It is striking how two different speakers can imbue the same sentence with entirely different types of utterance. This shows that the invasive, altering power to configure lies in *how* something is said. Analogously, two viewers perform two different acts from different positions and points of view. The way the act is performed is more important than what is seen. The fundamental bipolarity of seeing between response and spontaneity only becomes comprehensible by being carried out. When the performance of perception produces something to which the viewer reacts at the same time, then even an epistemic procedure such as identifying an object for the purpose of orientation can no longer be regarded as neutral recognition. The way seeing is practiced expresses a stylistic power of articulation by which the mode of execution determines what is seen. In this sense, the configuring act of organisation achieved by seeing is a formulation or reformulation of the matter-of-fact seen.

The difficulty of determining what style is in individual cases, the degree to which style is ineffable in the Wittgensteinian sense, is not relevant to the present theory of seeing. What is decisive is rather that the concept of style is not merely a nominal instrument for ordering types and periods within the diversity of expression, but rather is necessary to understanding the performative mode of an act of formulation. Style cannot be external to what it formulates, cannot be subtracted or added-on as a facultative, rhetorical flourish. The discussion of the so-called innocent eye demonstrated that the way we see cannot be a veil thrown over a 'neutral' perceptual content. Selectivity and diversity in seeing need to be explained by differences in the style of perception to the extent to which seeing is an act of formulation.

According to Humboldt's famous dictum, language is the "constitutive organ of thought. The intellectual activity, through and through mental, through and through inner, and, in a certain sense, passing without leaving a trace, becomes externally perceptible to the senses through sound in speech" (Humboldt 1973, p. 45). Analogously, if perception is to be understood as the constitutive organ of seeing, this process of constitution is in turn imperceptible to the other senses. If the performative character of seeing consists in a power of expression similar to formulation and presentation and determined by style, the question is how to subject it to reflection. The appropriate medium for getting at this may be visual art. A painter's viewpoint and seeing style materialise as visible objectifications when manifested in her painting style. As Konrad Fiedler has noted, every painting is an "act of seeing continued into the visible" (Fiedler 1991). H. Bahr refers to the history of painting as a history of styles of seeing (Bahr 1996, p. 117). If this is true, pictorial seeing should teach us something about the picture-making powers of seeing.

2.3 Iconic Seeing and Seeing Art

The style of a pictorial representation, as a particular way to show and to see, brings out the object in its unmistakable uniqueness. Style is recognisable at first glance without being exactly determinable. Picasso's and Matisse's flower vases differ so eminently in respect to style as to be unique, incomparable objects. In the history of art, style is the way of representing that is characteristic of a time and an artist, her unmistakable 'handwriting,' colouring and overwriting everything she sees and shows. According to H. Wölfflin in his analysis of style, "the essential character of a style"[11] (Wölfflin 1950) can be recognised "in the drawing of a mere nostril." Style adheres to a representation both visible and invisible and is equally significant for the representation as for the thing represented. It rises to the surface of the representation but cannot itself become an object of representation. Both a painter's individual style and stylistic features common to a period or genre generate unmistakable particularities, directed, as Luhmann once lucidly put it, not "to something better but rather something different" (Luhmann 1986, p. 634)—that is, toward ways of seeing that are of equal value.

The image occurs here twice: as representation and as what is represented. Representations show whatever they show in an idiosyncratic, characteristic style.

Richard Wohlheim has coined the term 'twofoldness' (Wollheim 1980) for pictorial representation's reflexive, doubled way of occurring. Pictures are *tableaux* and *images*, iconic medium and iconic subject. Within the pictorial medium the doubling occurs twice; as the duplicity of the representational medium—paint and brushwork—and the object represented.

[11]Wölfflin speaks explicitly of a "history of seeing" that together with period influence is responsible for the style of an epoch.

The twofold nature of the picture is repeated in its observation. Seeing something *in something*—that is, seeing what is represented in the representation—is necessarily a twofold act of attention. Attention is dual or divided as far as it is directed to the twofoldness of tableau and image. It can divide by alternating between the motif and the way it is represented.

Gombrich stresses that such divided attention can never simultaneously focus on both things, but rather alternates between the two acts of attention, as in picture puzzles (Gombrich 1960, p. 6). This means that seeing art entails a 'blindness' that alternates between the medium and what is mediated.[12] This is certainly true. But it is irrelevant in the present context whether we see either the one or the other or whether one runs on subliminally while we see the other. There is a different issue at stake for the question of seeing as (performative) practice. Within a finite image surface, an infinite image space becomes visible; something is seen *as* something else, the imaginative and imaginary character of which opens up infinite possibilities of interpretation. Iconic seeing must accept invention if it is to disclose the pictured (and later we will see that the case is similar when we see other persons). Iconic seeing doubles or splits into perceiving and imagining. Against Goodman's semiotic theory of the image, Michael Podro describes this splitting, when he asserts that "imagining and seeing" (Podro 1998, p. 27) cannot be separated from one another in seeing art works. There remains much to be said on the connection between seeing, representing and imagining. For the time being, suffice it to say that the as-structure of the image must be realised by an as-structure of seeing, by a *seeing something as something in something else* that must maintain constant relations to imagination.

2.4 Shown Seeing

It has been established that the twofoldness consists not only in the double visibility of the picture as object and as representation of an object, but it also recurs internally; the representation itself doubles or splits into *what* is shown and *how* it is shown—that is, in a represented *what* and a representing *how*. What is represented depends as much on the media and materials

[12] Gottfried Boehm (2001) has described something similar for seeing of the whole and parts in pictures. A focus on details is necessarily blind to the image as a whole. Conversely, a seeing that takes in the whole surface at once necessarily overlooks details of figures, brushwork and so on.

of the representation as on the artist's painting style and the capacities of the age to represent reality aesthetically. Painted images represent not only what an artist saw but how she saw it.

For A. Danto, a "main office of art" is "to represent the world [...] in such a way as to cause us to view it with a certain attitude and with a special vision" (Danto 1981, p. 167). By comparison, I want to illustrate such special ways of seeing that artworks open up. This should support the claims made above on the connection between style and way of seeing. In the 1460s, the Renaissance painters Andrea Mantegna and his brother-in-law Giovanni Bellini, both made renderings of the theme of Christ on the Mount of Olives (Figs. 1 and 2). The date is controversial, so there is no conclusive evidence as to which work was made earlier.

Although the compositions as a whole are extremely similar, the painters present very different views. Bellini's early work unifies the pictorial space with a realistic, warm light. This corresponds to a specifically Venetian and modern approach to images in which colours are treated as symbolical only in a limited sense. Colour is here chiefly a quality of light and of empirical

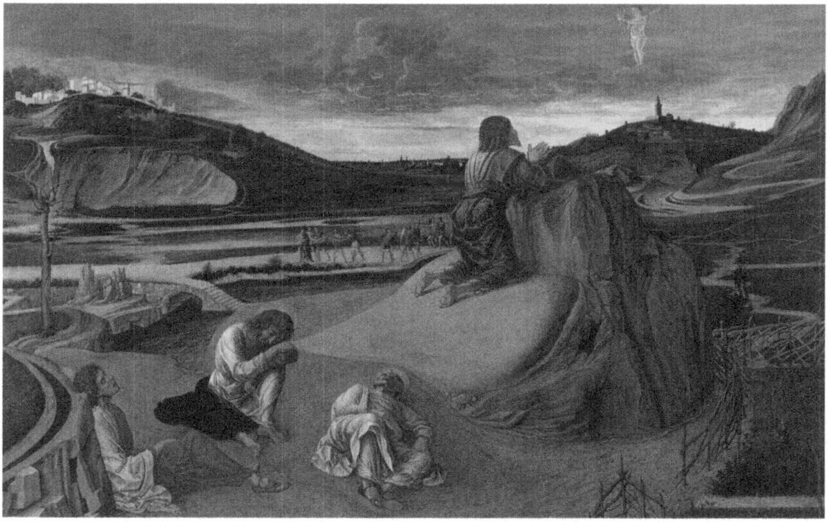

Fig. 1 Giovanni Bellini, *The Agony in the Garden*, ca. 1460, National Gallery London

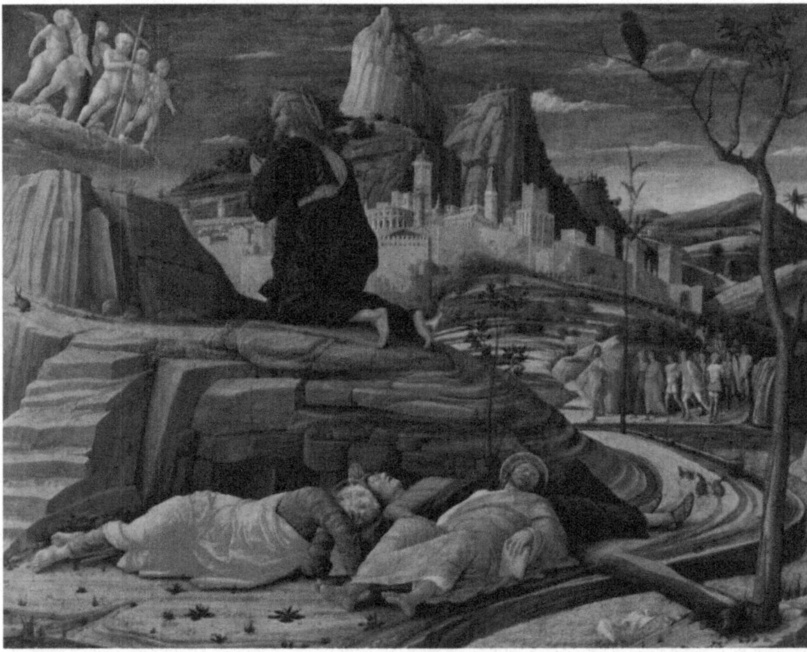

Fig. 2 Andrea Mantegna, *The Agony in the Garden*, ca. 1460, National Gallery London

reality (Huse 1972). Bellini avoids hard contours. Even the stone surface on which Christ is kneeling is soft and pliable.

By contrast, Mantegna's sharp, graphic line emphasises the monumentality and plasticity of the figure of Christ, starkly set off from the background. He piles up rock formations into a structure obstructing the view into the distance. The significantly darker colours adhere to the bodies, further separating the figures from one another, in contrast to Bellini's unifying, moody colouration. In opposition to his brother-in-law's use of tectonics, Mantegna's composition resists the Western convention of reading from left to right. Read in this way, it is dominated by a descending diagonal vector, whereas Bellini's lines lead the gaze upwards.

In this way, the two painters provide very different images of Christ, which can be interpreted as different understandings of God and religion. Without needing to commit to an interpretation, it can be said that the

Bellini painting is more a consolatory version of the Gethsemane theme as a theme of deliverance compared with Mantegna's, which emphasises human hopelessness. The story of the passion is thus differently accentuated. Is Christ the subject of meaningful suffering or the object of a story with no way out? Mantegna's image leaves it undecided as to whether God responds to the desperation of the harried/tormented Christ. The angels at the upper left bearing the attributes of the passion—the flagellation column, the vinegar sponge and the cross—may be Christ's vision of horror. Bellini's angels bearing the cup of the Eucharist, a reference to the religious meaning of the passion in the founding of the church, are more appropriate as God's answer.

Regardless of the particular interpretation, it is apparent that both images, despite their great similarity and comparability of content, demonstrate very different ways of seeing that content and these ways of seeing are primarily due to the style of representation. The images not only *show* the visible but *make* visible different possible ways of seeing it. This involves an act of translation comparable to that of metaphor, by virtue of constituting constellations that configure seeing. The style of representation begins already with an artist's style of perceiving, which makes the perceived visible both in its incomparability and its typicality. The way something is painted makes visible how it is seen.

In this respect, seeing exhibits a systematic proximity to showing. Both are fundamentally contingent on perspective, on a standpoint; the 'quid' is dependent on the 'quomodo'. It is impossible to see something neutrally because any allegedly neutral way of seeing is just a particular way of seeing—that is, a point of view. It is equally impossible to show something without introducing the expressivity of how it is shown. Just as the modal conditions of visibility, of the way in which something shows itself, determine how it appears and how it can be seen, so does the artist's style of representation and perception determine the ways the object shown can be taken up.

Showing and seeing, Deixis and Aisthesis, are determined by the same twofoldness and as-structure of the intentional viewpoint. The ability of a picture to show something and make it visible consists not so much in indexical showing as in an act of embodiment and realisation. What shows itself, presents itself as this particular thing and no other; for example, as a figure against a horizon and so on.

Showing is understood differently by analytic theorising than by phenomenology. Different levels of meaning can be distinguished among different acts of showing [Zeigen; signifying]; refering (deiknymi), demonstrating, illustrating and performing (Mersch 2002). There is a broad consensus that showing/signifying, as an aesthetic, analogous event, should be distinguished from discursive events.[13] This is a further indication that seeing cannot be regarded as a propositional act, but rather must be understood in its twofoldness as an aisthetic-aesthetic standpoint opened towards the polyvalent apparition of the world. Seeing can neither be as univalent as a statement, nor is the visible ever a determined, identical given. Rather, seeing must proceed analogically.

2.5 *Ethos and Habitus*

If it is admitted that the *how*, a painter's style of seeing, is to such a degree constitutive of the *what*, of the thing signified, then the connection can now be more precisely formulated between seeing and personal ways of seeing, and it can be determined which representative forces operate in each act of seeing. It is precisely this Janus-faced character specific to pictorial representation that we rediscover in seeing, inasmuch as seeing is fundamentally an act. Perspective determines what something can be shown as, making seeing more than just receptivity. Seeing determines the form of the seen and the development of a point of view. Just as the duplicity of a representational *what* and a modal *how* is constitutive for any form of iconicity, so too is it characteristic of the iconic and sense-making possibilities of seeing. For this reason, we can go so far as to attribute to seeing expressive qualities or a faculty of signification comparable to spoken expression. Seeing shows something by making something visible in a particular way.

The iconicity of seeing is a way of representing the seen that determines how something presents itself to me, as well as which ways of seeing and points of view I can adopt toward it. However, in order to communicate these ways of seeing to others, or to bring them to my own awareness, I need to treat them as lingual or reflective objects, as imperfect and incomplete this treatment may be. But even when this consciousness comes about only rarely, and can never succeed entirely, something is gained by making the

[13] See L. Wittgenstein (2001), N. Goodman (1976) and G. Abel (1999).

iconicity of seeing clear. Otherwise we could not understand the capacity of the senses for world disclosure.

It should by now have become clear that the representative style is not purely aesthetic, but deeply bound up with ethical qualities. To quote Danto again: "The structure of a style is like the structure of a personality [...] Learning to recognise a style is like learning to recognise a person's touch or his character" (Danto 1983, p. 207).

Any discussion of the morality of seeing will show that we can speak of an ethos of the viewer in the etymological ambiguity of the term: the way a person stands towards the world in her character and her habits. Normative inclinations to perceive things in certain ways and not others, as well as attitudes and habits, are a part of seeing. Acts of perception manifest a basic stance towards the world consisting of evaluative dispositions and ingrained ways of behaving and appearing.

With reference to Bourdieu's concept of praxis, this disposition can be spoken of as a habitus, which also involves style in an ethico-aesthetic sense.[14] A habitus is an agent's basic attitude within practice and as a formative force "une force *formatrice* d'habitude"[a *formative* force of habits] (Bourdieu 1974, p. 147), and as a dispositive independent of personality, which manifests stylistically in all action and speech. Such an individual disposition also informs habitual ways of seeing. The habitus is both conventional and individual, rooted in individual conditioning by life history, in experience and practice. It is the source of innovative divergence from collective norms of seeing. Habitus seeps into corporeal disposition, becomes apparent in gait, comportment, gesture and facial expression.

These are the basic dispositional prerequisites for the style, ethos and habitus of seeing, universally determining of the way we disclose the world in perception.

References

Abel, Günter. 1999. *Sprache, Zeichen, Interpretation*. Frankfurt a.M.: Suhrkamp.

Arendt, Hannah. 1959. *The Human Condition*. New York. Doubleday Anchor Books.

[14]Sociologists have long considered substituting the concept of lifestyle for the class model of society. See S. Hradil (1987). Hartmut Lüdtke (1989) has elucidated the distinctions to be gained by milieu-specific aesthetic preferences of everyday self-display.

Bahr, Hermann. 1996. From Expressionism. In *Art in Theory 1900-1990*, ed. Charles Harrison. Cambridge: Wiley-Blackwell.
Bergson, Henri. 2004. *Matter and Memory*. Mineola: Dover Publications.
Boehm, Gottfried (ed.). 2001. Repräsentation – Präsentation – Präsenz. In *Homo pictor*, 3–13. Leipzig: Saur.
Bourdieu, Pierre. 1974. *Architecture gothique et pensée scholastique*. Paris: Seuil.
Bryson, Norman. 1983. *Vision and Painting: The Logic of the Gaze*. New Haven: Yale University Press.
Butler, Judith. 1988. Performative Acts and Gender Constitution: An Essay in Phenomenology and Feminist Theory. *Theatre Journal* 40.4: 519–531.
Crutchfield, Richard S. et al. (eds.). 1982. *Elements of Psychology*. New York: A. Knopf.
Danto, Arthur. 1981. *The Transfiguration of the Commonplace*. Cambridge: Harvard University Press.
Danto, Arthur. 1983. *The Transfiguration of the Commonplace*. Cambridge: Harvard University Press.
Davidson, Donald. 2001. *Essays on Actions and Events: Philosophical Essays*. Oxford: Oxford University Press.
Fiedler, Konrad. 1991. *Schriften zur Kunst*. Munich: Fink.
Foerster, Heinz von. 1985. *Sicht und Einsicht*. Braunschweig: Vieweg+Teubner.
Frank, Manfred. 1990. *Stil in der Philosophie*. Stuttgart: Reclam.
Gehlen, Arnold. 1966. *Der Mensch*, 157–180. Frankfurt: Athenäum.
Gibson, James. 1966. *The Senses Considered as Perceptual Systems*. Boston, MA: Houghton Mifflin.
Gibson, James. 1986. *The Ecological Approach to Visual Perception*. Hillsdale: Routledge.
Goldstein, E. Bruce. 2002. *Sensation and Perception*. Pacific Grove, CA: Wadsworth.
Gombrich, Ernst. 1960. *Art and Illusion*. Princeton: Princeton University Press.
Goodman, Nelson. 1976. *Languages of Art: An Approach to a Theory of Symbols*. Indianapolis: Bobbs-Merrill.
Hart Nibbrig, Christiaan Lukas. 1994. Was heißt Darstellen? In *Was heißt Darstellen?*, ed. Christiaan Lukas Hart Nibbrig, 7–14. Frankfurt a.M.: Suhrkamp.
Hradil, Stefan. 1987. *Sozialstrukturanalyse in einer fortgeschrittenen Gesellschaft. Von Klassen und Schichten zu Lagen und Milieus*. Opladen: Leske + Burdrich.
Humboldt, Wilhelm von. 1973. *Schriften zur Sprache*. Stuttgart: Reclam.
Huse, Norbert. 1972. *Studien zu Giovanni Bellini*. Berlin: de Gruyter.
Kant, Immanuel. 2000. *Critique of the Power of Judgment*. Cambridge: Cambridge University Press.
Kertscher, Jens, and Mersch, Dieter (eds.). 2003. *Performativität und Praxis*. Munich: Fink.

Kolesch, Doris, and Krämer, Sybille (eds.). 2006. *Stimme*. Frankfurt a.M.: Suhrkamp.
Krämer, Sybille (ed.). 2004. *Performativität und Medialität*. Munich: Fink.
Lichtenberg, Georg Ludwig. 1984. *Sudelbücher*. Frankfurt a.M.: Insel Verlag.
Lüdtke, Hartmut. 1989. *Expressive Ungleichheit*. Opladen: Leske + Burdrich.
Luhmann, Niklas. 1986. Das Kunstwerk und die Selbstreproduktion der Kunst. In *Stil*, ed. Hans Ulrich Gumbrecht et al., 623–626. Frankfurt a.M.: Suhrkamp.
Lyotard, Jean-François. 1988. *The Differend: Phrases in Dispute*. Minneapolis: University of Minnesota Press.
MacIntyre, Alasdair. 2007. *After Virtue: A Study in Moral Theory*. Notre Dame: University of Notre Dame Press.
McGinn, Collin. 1999. *The Mysterious Flame*. New York: Basic Books.
Merleau-Ponty, Maurice. 1962. *Phenomenology of Perception*. London: Routledge.
Merleau-Ponty, Maurice. 1964. The Film and the New Psychology. In *Sense and Non-Sense*, 48–59. Evanston: Northwestern University Press.
Merleau-Ponty, Maurice. 1993. Indirect Language and the Voices of Silence. In *The Merleau-Ponty Aesthetics Reader: Philosophy and Painting*. Evanston: Northwestern University Press.
Mersch, Dieter. 2002. *Was sich zeigt*. Munich: Fink.
Mitchell, William John Thomas. 1986. *Iconology: Image, Text, Ideology*. Chicago: University of Chicago Press.
Mühleis, Volkmar. 2005. *Kunst im Sehverlust*. Munich: Fink.
Podro, Michael. 1998. *Depiction*. New Haven: Yale University Press.
Proust, Marcel. 1993. *In Search of Lost Time, Vol. VI: Time Regained*. New York: Modern Library.
Rosenberg, Rainer. 2003. Stil. In *Ästhetische Grundbegriffe*, Vol. 5, 641–664. Stuttgart: Metzler.
Saussure, Ferdinand de. 1976. *Cours de linguistique générale*. Paris: Payout.
Schmitz, Hermann. 1967. *Der leibliche Raum*. Bonn: Bouvier.
Sturma, Dieter. 1997. *Philosophie der Person*. Paderborn: Schöningh.
Sturma, Dieter. 2005. Die Selbstverhältnisse der Person. *Journal für Psychologie* 13.3: 240–254. Göttingen: Vandenhoeck & Ruprecht.
Weiskrantz, Lawrence. 1986. *Blindsight: A Case-Study and Implications*. Oxford: Oxford University Press.
Wirth, Uwe (ed.). 2002. *Performanz*. Frankfurt a.M.: Suhrkamp.
Wittgenstein, Ludwig. 2001. *Tractatus logico-philosophicus*. London: Routledge.
Wölfflin, Herinrich. 1950. *Principles of Art History*. New York: Dover Publications.
Wollheim, Richard. 1980. Seeing-as, Seeing-in and Pictorial Representation. In *Art and Its Objects*, 205–226. Cambridge: Cambridge University Press.
Wulf, Christoph, and Zirfas, Jörg (eds.). 2005. *Ikonologie des Performativen*. Munich: Fink.

CHAPTER 5

In Seeing Beyond Seeing

For a performative theory of perception as practice, seeing and the activities of thinking, interpreting and judging emerge as mediations between general rules and individual possibilities for divergence from those rules. The dense, occasionally insoluble nexus between sight and insight—as well as between seeing and ways of seeing—is closely bound up with the active character and its transformative capacities. Ways of seeing begin with the modal qualities of a particular way of seeing, which, influenced by sensory presence as well as absence makes seeing a plastic act that is both formed and formative.

Yet the relation between the visual and the mental still needs to be clarified. How and when does sight become insight? I want to introduce this new problem in the light of two philosophical positions from the twentieth century (Rentsch 2003): in his Philosophical Investigations, the later Wittgenstein explored the limits of the concept of seeing. Heidegger addressed seeing as a basic mode of Dasein. What Wittgenstein refers to as aspect-seeing is in Heidegger "articulate interpretation" (Heidegger 1996, §32, p. 140). Both are opposed to an ontology of fully present (preexisting) things and meanings.

Appended to these considerations, the second part of this chapter will attempt to reformulate the relation between seeing and ways of seeing, sensibility and sense making, as a relation of the visible to the invisible. This effort is guided by the assumption, first, that seeing has a world-disclosing quality analogous to that of language and, second, that this is

E. Schuermann, *Seeing as Practice*, Performance Philosophy,
https://doi.org/10.1007/978-3-030-14507-1_5

the case because there is a part of seeing that transcends seeing itself. Simple experiments in the psychology of perception (Goldstein 2002, p. 77ff.) demonstrate that imagination must inhere in seeing, for example, in order to account for the completion of incomplete visual information in seeing. The more an act of perception involves imagination, the more we need a concept of imagination specific to perception. If imagination, expectation, completion and interpretation enter into the practice of perception, it follows that something not sensibly present and therefore non-visible is mixed into the visible. The finding that seeing always occurs around the difference between the sensible and the intelligible, actuality and latency, leads to a concept of the invisible that includes everything that seeing owes to other acts of consciousness, expectation and memory—that is, the supplements of interpretation, will and opinion. Instead of speaking of the invisible, which may sound suspiciously metaphysical, the term 'non-actual perceptions' could be employed. Strawson employs such terms when describing the involvement of imagination in perception (Strawson 1970, p. 41) to indicate that not only are things present seen but that perception refers to things already seen, things customary and remembered, desired and believed. The imaginary character of these influences will be discussed separately in the chapter on imagination. Seeing as a world-disclosing practice is not a matter of cognition alone, but that desire, hope and fear influence seeing, is a point to be treated on its own. In the meantime, suffice it to say that perception maintains an uninterrupted relation to the mind.

1 Sight and Insight—Seeing and Ways of Seeing

The sense of sight has a specific capacity for freedom that clearly consists in its proximity to processes of understanding, of thought and of interpretation. It is often impossible to specify which part of seeing is the sensory part in the narrow sense, or when an act of attention becomes judgement, and what is the limit of perception. In order to be able to see that my child is growing up or is angry with me, it does not suffice to postulate sensory immediate givens. Nevertheless, this is still a case of seeing rather than hearing or dreaming. The child's grown-up demeanour and its furrowed brow are sensually perceivable properties of its visibility, which are unrecognisable without sight. This type of sight is literally insight. Merleau-Ponty is therefore justified in claiming there is "no seeing without thinking." Inversely, it is not enough "to think in order to see" (Merleau-Ponty 1964b, p. 175).

The visual and the mental appear to be inseparably interwoven in practice and can only be separated in theoretical description.

1.1 Wittgenstein's Aspect-Seeing

With reference to the famous drawing that can be seen as a rabbit or as a duck,[1] Wittgenstein describes aspect seeing as "half visual experience, half thought" (Wittgenstein 1986, Part 2, p. 168). Aspect seeing is a semantic 'seeing as.' I see something *as* something, namely the figure as a rabbit or as a duck. I do not see both meanings in the figure as I would see geographies in cloud formations, because I cannot see the drawing as something amorphous without recognising one of the other two figures. There are only two possible ways to see the image: R or D. The amphiboly from one to the other is constitutive of aspect seeing. There is a noteworthy correspondence here with the seeing of representation. When we see an actress represent someone—for example, Greta Garbo as Mata Hari—this seeing involves a different characteristic of aspect seeing. The image of the face stays the same but the way we see it changes.

Over and above the psychology of perception, double images and puzzle pictures are relevant to the relation between seeing and interpreting, perceiving and imagining. Wittgenstein asks: "Do I really see something different each time, or do I only interpret what I see in a different way? I am inclined to say the former. But why?" (Wittgenstein 1986, Part 2, p. 181).

This is another case of it being impossible to unequivocally determine the relation between thinking and seeing. Wittgenstein's characterisation of seeing as a state is countered by his own reflections. Indeed, he appears uncertain of his case. If he is inclined to say that he actually sees something different each time, then seeing must also be doing—a doing in which the attribution of meaning is an integral part. The act of attribution is a procedure that cannot be divorced from the act of perception. This severance would be required in order to distinguish an independent perceptual state

[1] Wittgenstein knew this figure from the works of the American psychologist Joseph Jastrow, who publishes his reflections on it in 1899. The double image was first printed in 1892 in the weekly 'Fliegende Blätter.' See Kihlstrom (2018).

from an operation of thought involving inference.[2] Aspect seeing is therefore a good example for the indivisibility of perception and sense making. Whether I see the marks as the contours of a rabbit or a duck is not a question of posterior judgement. Rather, the visual apprehension is given simultaneously with the impression of this or that figure. Aspect seeing is thus similar to iconic seeing. We "*see* it as we *interpret* it" (Wittgenstein 1986, Part 2, p. 165).

The way seeing is dependent on context is also manifest in the R–D example. If the image is viewed for the first time within a series of other rabbit images, it is difficult to recognise the duck's head, because the context has conditioned the expectation that further rabbits will appear.

The picture puzzle is an especially striking example of a permanent feature of seeing: adoption of perspectives from which something appears as x rather than as y. Presumably, with practically everything we see, we have several options concerning what we see it as. Things give occasion to a variety of views. The way it appears need not be in any way illusory but is rather the self-justified and unavoidable way in which it shows itself; never of course the whole but rather a partial aspect of all that it could also otherwise be.

There does not exist an indefinite number of possible interpretations of the figure. Seeing it as a rabbit or duck are both equally given ways of seeing that are not arbitrary. The small irregularity that would be the rabbit's mouth is an important detail that would be meaningless if we could not see the figure as a rabbit. Without this detail, it would be difficult to see the rabbit at all, instead of just seeing the duck. This suggests the evocative power with which the visible determines perception.

By seeking criteria for what could be called 'genuine seeing,' Wittgenstein encounters the limits of language use:

> "But this isn't seeing!"——"But this is seeing!"—It must be possible to give both remarks a conceptual justification.

[2] In his commentary to Wittgenstein's reflections, Thorsten Jantschek (1997, p. 311) writes that thought involves making an assumption beyond the seen. If it were so simple, the seen would have to be susceptible to a description independent of interpretation: "When we interpret something we build an assumption, a hypothesis about something given." However, no image exists independently of being interpreted as either a rabbit or a duck. Hence we are better served with "the insight that thinking and seeing are always already related to one-another and this relationship manifests in seeing-as" (ibid., p. 319).

> But this is seeing! In what sense is it seeing? (Wittgenstein 1986, Part 2, p. 203)

The difficulties are once again related to theoretical distinctions made by a language of description. In order to describe this type of seeing-as, we need to presuppose a basic sense-perception level, although the whole gist of the talk of aspect seeing is the inseparability of the visual and the mental. They are both separate and not separate. They must be separate because acts of responsive apprehension are generally distinguishable from acts of logical deduction or narrative interpretation. Yet they must be at the same time non-separate, because my perception is not of raw sensory material, but is always already meaningfully organised.

The constitutive proximity of seeing and understanding has also been referred to as the way visual perception is charged with theory, meaning the inclination of the perceiver to see in terms of theoretical insights and beliefs. Ludwig Fleck's early investigation of thought style as preparedness for directed perception (Fleck 1981, p. 99) is foundational in this regard. Wittgenstein makes similar use of the term 'Denkstil,'[3] style of thinking, as a method of examination and justification (Schulte 1990, p. 61), which begins with a way of seeing (Nordmann 2003). Thomas Kuhn describes abrupt paradigm shifts in the sciences as seeing-as. After a scientific revolution, the world is seen as something else. "What were ducks in the scientist's world before the revolution are rabbits afterwards" (Kuhn 1970, p. 111). Accordingly, seeing something differently, in this context, is seeing it within the framework of a different theory.[4]

1.2 Heidegger's Interpretation

Heidegger has elucidated the inseparability of thinking and seeing as interpretation. He writes:

> But if any perception of useful things at hang always understands and interprets them, letting them be circumspectly encountered as something, does

[3] L. Wittgenstein: "How much we are doing is changing the style of thinking and how much I'm doing is changing the style of thinking and how much I'm doing is persuading people to change their style of thinking" (Wittgenstein 2007, p. 28).

[4] Judith Genova (1995) reads Wittgenstein's whole thinking as methodically applied aspect-seeing, to the purpose of seeing otherwise than usual.

> this not then mean that initially something merely objectively present is experienced which then is understood *as* a door, *as* a house? That would be a misunderstanding of the specific disclosive function of interpretation. (Heidegger 1996, p. 140).

'Mere seeing' already "contains the structure of interpretation," everything else is uncomprehending 'staring' (ibid., p. 140). Against the myth of the given, Heidegger asserts that the notion of grasping 'free of the as' is in no way an original form of perception on which comprehending seeing builds, but rather an artificially derived privative form of the latter. Interpretation is not the posterior bestowing of a meaning on something 'in itself' meaningless but, rather, interpretation of the relational whole [*Bewandtnisganzheit*] of understanding the world.

Like any form of world disclosure, interpretation is an act of understanding with circular presuppositions. Interpreting something as something is grounded in the anticipation of a certain basic conception, which the interpretation has always already (finally or at least preliminarily) decided upon. "Interpretation is never a presuppositionless grasping of something previously given" (ibid., p. 141). Pre-understanding denotes the hermeneutic structure of a specific, culturally and historically conditioned disposition to understand. To invoke a 'presented' is to invoke (in Heidegger's example, the text being interpreted) "nothing else than the self-evident, undisputed prejudice [*Vormeinung*] of the interpreter" (ibid.).

Comparable to Wittgenstein's thought-styles conditioned by a worldview, the hermeneutic conception of pre-understanding decides how, and as what, something visible can be seen. The visible is always only visible under the conditions of the "fore-structure of understanding and the as-structure of interpretation" (ibid.). The as-structure of understanding is equally due to directed consciousness that perceives something as something, and due to the visible itself showing itself as-something, in the light of a situation and against the background of invisible framing factors constituted by history, culture and society.

Which view I can assume depends on the assumption of points of view on the part of pre-understanding. The circumspection (*Umsicht*) of care (*besorgen*), the hindsight (*Rücksicht*) of caring for, far from being mere figures of speech, express existential ways of seeing, syntheses of thinking and outlook. What Heidegger refers to as interpretive seeing is a form of aisthetic world disclosure consisting in hermeneutic acts in which we apply the familiar to the novel, frame it in a new horizon, apprehend present things and complement them by the addition of imaginative invention. It is as such both receptive and projective.

1.3 The Inevitability of Metaphor

So far, we have found that Heidegger and Wittgenstein agree that thinking and seeing (and, with it, perceptual reference to what is present as well as to what is absent) exhibit a closeness that borders on indistinguishability. Just like, for Wittgenstein, thought-style, worldview and form of life prefigure what can be seen and experienced, so for Heidegger, it is the relational whole (*Bewandtnisganzheit*) of pre-understanding and interpreting being-in-the world that contextually endow perception with meaning. In framing matters thus, both philosophers can be seen to criticise representational notions of thinking as well as perceiving.

As in the example of Petrarch from the Introduction Chapter, seeing shows itself to be a two-faceted act turned simultaneously towards consciousness and towards the world, with the viewer turning out to be simultaneously bios theoretikos *and* bios praktikos. Thus, at the core of seeing there is something that extends beyond seeing and the visible itself.

In many languages, the connection between sight and insight is compounded in words like *Gesichtspunkt, Ansicht, Überblick, point de vue, considerazione*. What is expressed here is the unity of that which the thinking of the given divides up, namely the simultaneity of an act of visual perception directed at both the visible and the invisible. The entire metaphor of understanding as seeing suggests this inextricability of the sensory and the mental. The vocabulary of acts of understanding and thought points, in many languages, to a visuality of cognition and to an intelligibility in perception. This begins presumably with the Greek term θεωρία for a seeing that is at once sensory and mental. It continues with the Latin perspicere, the French 'voir' in 'sa-voir,' with the double meaning of the Italian 'guardare,' with the meanings to guard and to take care of, and with the English 'I see what you mean.' In the Greek, the perfect of εἴδω 'I see' is οἶδα, 'I have seen' and is equivalent in meaning to 'I know.' Knowledge is construed as the result of having seen. This explains the weight of eyewitness accounts and visual demonstrations. The visuality of processes of knowledge acquisition and understanding expressed in this use of language is a forceful expression of what may be called the theory-laden nature of the sense of sight. Far beyond figurative speech, it articulates a systematic connection between sight, insight, understanding, interpretation, opinion formation, conviction and knowledge.

With Blumenberg, seeing can thus be designated as an absolute metaphor, and that the verba videndi stand in where logic fails (Blumenberg 2010, p. 3) This befalls thought where it attempts to explain the relation between sight and insight. No well-defined 'literal' term for seeing can be isolated from metaphorical talk of seeing. Rather, the figurative speech indicates an unavoidable problem, the unavoidability of which demands attention[5] since it signals that reducing the sense of sight to perception is to artificially isolate only one part of seeing from a holistic act. The metaphorical nature of the term itself offers a way to render seeing manifest. To speak of seeing 'with other eyes,' of overlooking or oversight, of ways of looking at things, is not merely a way of speaking that could be translated into a clearer language or replaced with non-pictorial terms. Rather, seeing is in the 'mantic'[6] field of connotations of understanding; it is the literal movement of in-sight, which cannot be grasped purely aisthetically or mentally. It is an aisthetic way of world disclosure, the aesthetic and imaginary ramifications of which require investigation in individual cases. For a holistic understanding of perception, to speak of 'pro-viding' or 'seeing through' something, these are not merely figurative descriptions. Nor are they basic or simple perceptual acts, since the assumption of such acts is itself mixed up with a misleading use of terms. Such activities are at once aisthetic and epistemic, bound to the use of the eyes but without being reducible to these.

There are isolated cases of the use of metaphors of seeing. In order to 'see' what someone means, I do not need to see something before me. The act or state of 'respecting' someone is not itself an act of perception. Yet in the context of the many-layered interconnections of the aisthetic and the mental, such relatively clear-cut cases are rather more the exception than the rule.

It is much more common to *see* that someone wants to speak, or how the way someone is looked up to hinges on the way she looks, for example.

[5] Ralf Konersmann (1991) has played through similar notions regarding the metaphor of the mirror. The fugitiveness of the term makes it an appropriate image of the intangibility of a subjectivity that eludes itself.

[6] On the uninterrupted relation between understanding and interpretation, see W. Hogrebe (1996).

The cultural semantics of light as a synonym for truth, invoked by both mystics and rationalists, hang together within this whole of the visual and the mental. There is practically no 'literal' talk of light, since the effect of light on the eyes is the basic physical enabling condition of seeing. Such literal talk is in any case impossible without running into a history of terms that would conventionally be designated as metaphorical. In the Greek metaphor of light, light counts as the condition of insightful knowledge in both the figurative and literal senses. Light makes "being able to be seen and being able to see really possible," (Böhme 2000, p. 350) as G. Böhme explains with reference to the Platonic beginnings of the philosophy of light. Light is the joining medium that makes the visible and the faculty of seeing a mutual reality. Plato's sun of the good, light as the magic word of the Enlightenment, the lucidity of being, the likeness of the eyes to the sun, are all tangible and non-interchangeable images of the occidental tradition of thought, omnipresent thanks both to the semantics of both religion and the enlightenment. The light of the eyes renders transparent, evident; it is the principle of the capacity of sight and insight, a necessary medium of perception like space and time. The mystic view and rational insight, talk of the light of God and the light of reason, are founded on the assumption of truth as a type of light, which can be seen and observed, and a coincidence of seeing and understanding that is lost sight of in the theoretical analysis of cognition, and simply discarded in the assumption of a hierarchical ascension from perception, thinking and interpretation.

This cluster of terms is genuinely metaphorical in the sense that it cannot be translated back into a literal meaning and does not provide merely rhetorical ornamentation but rather discloses a relational whole.

It therefore appears both useful and obligatory to assume that it is not 'mere metaphor' when we say: something is provided for, we re-vise something, something is shown in a certain light, seen from certain points of view (Chladenius', '*Sehe-Punckte*' [viewpoints] [Chladenius 1742], formerly referred to as *Standpunkte* [standpoints] [Röttgers 1994]). Beyond these images, there is no authentic term for seeing. The process of perspectival seeing cannot be reduced to a univocal term.

Subsequently, and this is significant for the further development, seeing invisible things 'in the mind's eye'[7]—that is, seeing what can only be

[7] I avoid this expression as far as possible in order not to fall back into the division between physical and mental seeing. The point here is, however, to refer to a term responsible for the entire tradition of the idea of the given. It is indicative of the intricacies of the problem that

known or wished, is precisely not an exclusively mental activity but rather a hybrid of aesthetically and mentally occasioned ways of seeing. This view has gained support from analytic philosophy. Since 2002, the theorist of consciousness Colin McGinn has developed a similar approach with his notion of mindsight (McGinn 2004). While he follows Sartre in listing criteria for differentiating perceptions and images and assuming that they are not gradually, but fundamentally distinct, in the second chapter of his investigation he makes mention of 'the mind's eye,' which is not to be taken as metaphorical: "I shall argue, that [...] the phrase 'the mind's eye' is not metaphorical. It is literally true that we see with our mind" (McGinn 2004, p. 42). In the third chapter, he speaks of a hybrid of bodily ("a 'with the body' kind of seeing") and mental seeing, "imaginative seeing," which comprehends "the seeing of aspects, the seeing of pictures, and imagination-driven perceptual distortions" (McGinn 2004, p. 49). McGinn's argument revolves around its own point of departure in which he assumes a strict analytic division between perception and imagination. He is obliged to admit that the dichotomies collapse in practice, since imaginings possess visual properties and perceptions have pictorial properties that render them inseparable.

To reiterate the question posed at the outset of the chapter: it is necessary to describe the relation between the visual and the mental otherwise than in a model containing discrete steps, because a closer observation of the practice of seeing repeatedly and variously brings to light parts of seeing that go beyond seeing, i.e. thought, imagination, and interpretation.

If the seeing of aspects is not to be grasped in opposition to thought, it could be described as an 'analogical procedure' that, unlike logical thinking, does not urge toward 'differentiating the similar' but rather seeks, by means of comparison, to find 'similarity in difference' (Gabriel 1997, p. 370). As elucidated by G. Gabriel, analogical thinking seeks not definitions but instructive parallels. Whereas the thinking of identity suppresses the particular by subsuming it under the general, the analogous procedure attains knowledge by acquaintance of the particular and the singular. It consists in the constitution and discovery of characteristic aspects and meanings and thus displays a curious similarity to the way metaphor works in language. This will be developed more fully later on in the book.[8]

even authors like Sartre and McGinn use the term, although they postulate the cooperation of the mental and the visual in practice.

[8] See Sect. 1 in Chapter 7.

2 The Visible and the Invisible

What is the nature of the visible to which seeing must be open in order for something in the sensible to transcend itself?

The seemingly trivial finding that there must be something visible in order to be able to speak of seeing touches on what is in fact a complex question. It is difficult to determine more exactly the foundation of seeing. The problems begin with the fact that the visible is held to be an objective presence. If the visible were merely this flagrant objectivity, there would be no freedom to see in different ways. The visibility of the world, however, is not an unquestionable given but rather a mode of qualitative self-display and being-seen, nuanced by changes in perspective. If the world were to be understood as given objectively and independently of processes of apparition and perception, it would be unclear why it is capable of appearing differently. If it were an objective outer surface of things, their empirical appearance [aussehen; literally, out-seeing], then univocally determining the colour and form of things would present no difficulties. Neither can we say that everything capable of being seen is really seen, nor is what we overlook necessarily invisible. Which visible things are evocative enough to attract attention depends on so many framing factors that something within seeing always goes beyond seeing. The objective visible is thus just as mythical a creature as the innocent eye. Visible things may be classified as fascinating, enthralling, or boring, not in general, but only according to the particular case.

Among the various answers to the question of the relation between seeing and the visible, at least five concepts can be distinguished: interpretational, representational, correspondence/adequation, causal/motivational and dispositional. The general theoretical framework determines which answer is given. What follows concerns the concepts that assume a dispositional relation.

2.1 *Dispositive Instead of Referential*

Opponents of adequation theories of perception, such as Friedrich Nietzsche, vehemently deny that the reference of perception can be explained in terms of correspondence: "the correct perception—which would mean the full and adequate expression of an object in the subject—is something contradictory and impossible; for between two absolutely different spheres, as subject and object are, there is no causality, no correctness, and no expression, but most an aesthetic way of relating, by which I mean an allusive transference, a stammering translation into a quite different language. For which purpose a middle sphere und mediating force is certainly required" (Nietzsche 1999, p. 148). What is meant by aesthetic relation will be of interest to us later as the *art of seeing differently*.

The difficulty concerning the exact determination of reference results from the lack of an appropriate vocabulary for describing states of the world and the constitution of reality without falling back into disjunctions that overlook the processual connectedness of the I and the world. The question of the adequacy or correspondence of object relations is badly formulated[9] since it maintains the opposition between subject and object, fact and image.

Subsequently, what is required is a concept of the visible that is capable of explaining why the given is overlooked and why opinions can diverge about what is visible.

As J.-F. Lyotard writes, "In order to see, one oscillates between the current or actual and the possible by repeated pulsations" (Lyotard 1988, p. 45). The temporality of seeing and the visible means that there are continuously changing configurations of the 'see-able.' There must also be a dimension of possibility within the reality of the visible to which seeing relates as Ἐνέργεια to Εργον—that is, as an act in which and by which something is realised as its result. In agreement with Aristotle, it could be said that just as every reality is a development toward its other—for example, sleep is δυναμει δύναμαι [potential] waking—so too could the perceived world be the actualisation of the polyvalent see-able.

Real possibilities are distinguished in modal logic from the merely thinkable or dreamable (see Hartmann 2013). When from the indeterminate sphere of the potentially visible, the αισθητον Αίσθητόν, something determinate emerges, something that attracts attention; this is not explicable in a discrete ontology of a set of givens outside of any context, but rather at best as a changing configuration of possibilities of seeing. The relation between anticipation, already having seen, making present and interpreting could be specified as actualising possibilities that could also be actualised

[9]Mike Sandbothe (2001, p. 88) argues convincingly for this when he writes, "although realistic picture-copy theories and anti-realistic constructivist theories apply different criteria of adequation and presuppose different concepts of reality they remain in the same paradigm of representation aimed at correspondence."

differently. Within this model, perceptions actualise whatever is perceivable at that instant; this is also a mode of possibility not definitively determinable but rather one which contains an open spectrum of options of realisation.

Plato in the *Theaetetus* can be cited as providing just such a modalised concept of the visual. He opposes the "*power* of being *able to* be perceived" not to perception itself, but to the "*power* of being able to perceive" (Böhme 2000, p. 348). In the sun simile in the Politeia, Plato represents light as the third element in the triad of these two faculties whose interaction actualises a possibility of seeing in experience.

If this is the case, a horizon of latent and possible visibility overreaches whatever is actually being seen. A dimension of possibility structures the field of the visible in a similar way to the fields of space and time. The act of seeing is no more exhausted in what is seen than is the act of speech in what is spoken. The process of seeing is always informed by a surplus or an under-determination, the aesthetic and the anaesthetic (Welsch 1990).

If these considerations can be made more convincing still, we could assume that the visible and the viewer are essentially a mutually conditioned relation in which what is perceptible is evoked and motivated by what is *compossible* to the two at a given time in a socially shared world. This would explain the selective and interpretive character of perception as well as its invariables and agreements between subjects. This allows the visible to be not only 'objective' but also a dispositive element that occasions and enables perception.

2.2 Perception According to Merleau-Ponty

The French phenomenologist Maurice Merleau-Ponty is better qualified than anyone to provide a suitable concept of the non-actual, sensually absent, the merely possibly visible and the absolutely invisible. His unfinished late work, *Le Visible et l'invisible*[10] (Merleau-Ponty 1968), which appeared posthumously in 1964 and was translated into English in 1968, offers an abundance of considerations on the subject. I will not undertake a careful reconstruction of the speculative dimension of his notes,[11]

[10]Quotes from this edition, in the following abbreviated to VI.

[11]Merleau-Ponty's (1968, p. 139) meditations become speculative with the, in my opinion somewhat obscure, notion of the "chair"—flesh with which he attempts to define the common texture of the visible and the invisible. Flesh designates an "element" like water or air "between the spatio-temporal individual and the idea."

left unfinished at his death. His early work, *Phenomenology of Perception*, presents a multifaceted, insightful theory of physical perception (Schuermann 2000). Several of its main features will be sketched out and drawn upon. Additionally, the later discussion of the art of Paul Cézanne and William Kentridge will render the concept of the invisible significantly more concrete. The main purpose of this excursus is to come closer to the amphibolies of the invisible and the visible in seeing. In his search for the "extravagant consequences to which we are led when we take seriously, when we question, vision" (Merleau-Ponty 1968, p. 140), Merleau-Ponty works out a concept of seeing and visibility that—like his concept of practice—seeks to relinquish the subject-object dichotomy. He grasps seeing as a dialectical movement within the difference between the finite and the infinite, the sensory and the mental, without ever affixing it to one side.

His point of departure is the corporeality of the act of seeing. On the basis of a pre-predicative corporeal familiarity with the world as a pre-theoretical, meaningful context, he develops seeing as a corporeal affect—as touched touching. The sense of sight is thus not separated from the other senses, but is involved in an extremely dense interplay with them.

The sort of unchallenged relations of dominance described by Sartre do not occur in Merleau-Ponty's conception. "Immersed in the visible by his body, itself visible, the see-er does not appropriate what he sees; he merely approaches it by looking, he opens himself to the world" (Merleau-Ponty 1964b, p. 162). If we think in the categories of subject and object, according to Merleau-Ponty's invective against Sartre, there can be no encounter with the other.

By contrast, he understands the gaze as the "dehiscence of the seeing into the visible" (Merleau-Ponty 1968, p. 153), which disallows distance. He further objects that Sartre forgets the corporeal: "Vision is not the immediate relationship of the For Itself with the In Itself, and we are invited to redefine the seer as well as the world seen. The analytic of Being and Nothingness is the seer who forgets that he has a body" (ibid., p. 77).

In Merleau-Ponty's theory, the act of seeing is not dominated by a metaphysics of presence but is a seeing and see-able way of being in the world. His critique is directed less at the concept of presence than against the camera obscura model of the eye as the neutral receptor of sensations that itself does not affect the object it discloses. "Our fleshly eyes are already much more than receptors for light rays, colors, and lines" (Merleau-Ponty 1964b, p. 165). Perception has been falsely regarded by classical psychology as "a real deciphering of sense data by the intelligence" (ibid., p. 49). Perception is not mere "registering what the retinal stimuli prescribe but reorganizes these stimuli so as to re-establish the field's homogeneity. Broadly speaking, we should think of it not as a mosaic but as a system of configurations. Groups rather than juxtaposed elements are principal and primary in our perception" (Merleau-Ponty 1964a, p. 48). This holistic concept of perception goes against the reductionism of traditional psychology, where the latter presupposes "neutral sense data," which undergo posterior refinement into something intelligible.[12]

Merleau-Ponty's concept of seeing attempts to do justice to the alterity of the seen as a quality that resists appropriation. By this route, however, he does not escape the intentionality of seeing. Nevertheless, he suggests an alternative to the conception of seeing as a commanding overview, since "in the aerial view of the panorama, there can be no encounter with another" (Merleau-Ponty 1968, p. 77). To stress the aspect of encounter in seeing, he places in opposition to the panorama, the notion of chiasm, the overlap of the viewer and the viewed, a concept that undermines a one-sided determination. The look opens up views and these views "are not desultory—I do not look at a chaos, but at things—so that finally one cannot say if it is the look or if it is the things that command" (ibid., p. 133). The overlap can go so far that "we no longer know which sees and which is seen" (ibid., p. 139). The chiasm is a type of divided unity, as opposed to a simple coincidence (see Schuermann 2005).

The intertwinement of the visible and the invisible is also connected to this chiastic structure. It is a peculiarity of the visible to be "What this ultimately means is that the proper essence [le propre] of the visible is to have a layer [doublure] of invisibility in the strict sense, which it makes present as a certain absence" (Merleau-Ponty 1964b, p. 187). A significant part of this doubling is due to the surplus of possibility, which we have already encountered several times. The visible is always more and less than is actually seen. But the invisible is both more than this and different. It is noticeable on different levels: as deficit or surplus, as principally invisible and coincidentally unnoticed, as the blindness of seeing and perspectival

[12] B. Waldenfels (2000, p. 310) illustrates Merleau-Ponty's concept as follows: "Originary seeing is like a stone thrown into water, not a light bulb getting switched on." The image of circles cast in water is also used by Humboldt to explain the effect of speech, which seldom generates a single meaning but rather resonates in polyvalence (see Humboldt 1973, pp. 24, 58, and passim).

nuancing of the seen. It can be divided into a sensual and a non-sensual side. The knowledge I bring to the visible is itself non-sensual. In the art of Cézanne, in which Merleau-Ponty finds "a figured philosophy of vision—its iconography" (ibid., p. 168), knowledge of what the visible is must be suppressed in order to get closer to its *how*, to the way it is visible. In this way, according to Merleau-Ponty, painting can make something visible while at the same time preserving its enigma; that is, without conceptual identification: "Only the painter is entitled to look at everything without being obliged to appraise what he sees" (ibid., p. 161).

In all these cases, the invisible is a negative[13] that belongs to the essence of the visible as silence does to speech. More than the unseen and Husserl's 'das Unsichtige' (Husserl 1973), which is anticipated and pre-complemented, because the visible only ever appears in a given perspective, according to Merleau-Ponty, the invisible is a moment in the visible world that does not become visible from another viewpoint. The invisible is an essential dimension of absence in the present.

The visible gives rise to a perception that the viewer takes on according to her own preconditions. Neither of the two sides is fully free or fully determined. In this way, Merleau-Ponty arrives at a concept of perception with which he seeks to revise the ontology of the subject-object separation. Seeing mediates in such a way between consciousness and its object so as to connect the two in their separateness.

Merleau-Ponty's conception is eminently adaptable to a theory of seeing as practice due to the way it illuminates the meaningful simultaneity of production and response in the sense of sight. Where the general concept of practice implies sets of interconnections that cannot be reduced to a subject or an object, to freedom or determinacy, Merleau-Ponty's grasp of the practice of perception in particular entails a negative encircling of the peculiar hybrids that lie in the interval between the visible and the invisible.

By stressing the corporeality of the operation of seeing, its embeddedness in the whole of being-in-the-world is brought to bear on the issue. There is a shift away from the Wittgensteinian approach of reconstructing seeing pragmatically from within language use and forms of life. This shift does not strictly contradict Wittgenstein, but rather complements his ideas, adding and addressing an aspect that he mistakenly neglected.

[13]For the further implications of negativity in Merleau-Ponty's later work, see Gamm (1994).

2.3 *Figure and Ground*

Following on from these considerations, the relation between the visible and the invisible can be designated as a nexus of figure and ground. A figure comes into focus when the ground becomes unfocused. Conversely, in order to see the whole, the figure itself must be overlooked. The medium must become invisible if what it mediates is to be seen. The paradigm of transparency, the notion of painting as a window onto the world is based on this invisibility of the medium. A simple example for this interference between the visible and the invisible is reading. The reader must entirely overlook the optical apparition of black type on the white page in order to grasp the content. Just as the medium disappears behind the mediated, so too is seeing founded on partial invisibility.

The blind spot is thus productive, generates invisibility, against the background of which it is possible for something to appear *as something*. To perceiving the tree at the window as contoured, I need to make its surroundings recede. Inversely, gaining an overview of the whole entrains a loss of detail. Transparency is founded on opacity[14] and vice and versa.

The visible cannot be itself without its counterpart. The non-visible is a condition of the possibility of the visible in at least three senses: as the invisibility of the temporality of seeing; as the invisibility of spatial limits, in which the viewer is restricted to an excerpt; and as the invisibility of the viewers themselves, who do not see themselves seeing.

What perception occasions is only negatively nameable. But it is precisely for this reason that it cannot be depicted neutrally. The invisible—whether coincidentally overlooked, principally unseen or temporarily blocked—belongs not to another world, but is part of the visible itself.

References

Blumenberg, Hans. 2010. *Paradigms for a Metaphorology*. New York: Cornell University Press.

Böhme, Gernot. 2000. *Platons theoretische Philosophie*. Stuttgart: Metzler.

Chladenius, Johann Martin. 1742. *Einleitung zur richtigen Auslegung vernünftiger Reden und Schriften*. Leipzig: Buchhaus Stern-Verlag.

Fleck, Ludwik. 1981. *The Genesis and Development of a Scientific Fact*. Chicago: University of Chicago Press.

[14] Peter Geimer (2002) has described this state of affairs using the example of technical errors in photography, which undermine the paradigm established for the medium by Barthes.

Gabriel, Gottfried. 1997. Logisches und analogisches Denken. In *Sprache und Denken*, ed. Alex Burri, 370–384. Berlin: De Gruyter.
Gamm, Gerhard. 1994. *Flucht aus der Kategorie*. Frankfurt am Main: Suhrkamp.
Geimer, Peter (ed.). 2002. Was ist kein Bild? In *Ordnungen der Sichtbarkeit*, 313–341. Frankfurt am Main: Suhrkamp.
Genova, Judith. 1995. *Wittgenstein—A Way of Seeing*. New York and London: Routledge.
Goldstein, Bruce. 2002. *Sensation and Perception*. Pacific Grove: Wadsworth.
Hartmann, Nicolai. 2013. *Possibility and Actuality*. Berlin: De Gruyter.
Heidegger, Martin. 1996. *Being and Time*. Albany: State University of New York Press.
Hogrebe, Wolfram. 1996. *Erkenntnis und Ahnung*. Berlin: Akademie Verlag.
Humboldt, Wilhelm von. 1973. *Schriften zur Sprache*. Stuttgart: Reclam.
Husserl, Edmund. 1973. *Experience and Judgement*. Evanston: Northwestern University Press.
Jantschek, Thorsten. 1997. Bemerkungen zum Begriff des Sehen-als. In *Kritik des Sehens*, ed. Ralf Konersmann, 299–319. Leipzig: Reclam.
Kihlstrom, John F. 2018. *Joseph Jastrow and His Duck—Or Is It a Rabbit?* https://www.ocf.berkeley.edu/~jfkihlstrom/JastrowDuck.htm. Accessed 29 September 2019.
Konersmann, Ralf. 1991. *Lebendige Spiegel*. Frankfurt am Main: Fischer.
Kuhn, Thomas. 1970. *The Structure of Scientific Revolutions*. Chicago: University of Chicago Press.
Lyotard, Jean-Francois. 1988. *The Differend: Phrases in Dispute*. Minneapolis: University of Minnesota Press.
McGinn, Colin. 2004. *Mindsight: Image, Dream, Meaning*. Cambridge: Harvard University Press.
Merleau-Ponty, Maurice. 1964a. The Film and the New Psychology. In *Sense and Non-Sense*, 48–59. Evanston: Northwestern University Press.
Merleau-Ponty, Maurice. 1964b. Eye and Mind. In *The Primacy of Perception*, 159–190. Evanston: Northwestern University Press.
Merleau-Ponty, Maurice. 1968. T*he Visible and the Invisible*. Evanston: Northwestern University Press.
Nietzsche, Friedrich. 1999. On Truth and Lying in a Non-Moral Sense. In *The Birth of Tragedy and Other Writings*, 139–153. Cambridge: Cambridge University Press.
Nordmann, Alfred. 2003. "I Have Changed His Way of Seeing": Goethe, Lichtenberg and Wittgenstein. In *Goethe and Wittgenstein*, ed. Breithaupt, 91–110. Frankfurt am Main: Peter Lang Publishing.
Rentsch, Thomas. 2003. *Heidegger und Wittgenstein*. Stuttgart: Klett-Cotta.
Röttgers, Kurt. 1994. Der Standpunkt und die Gesichtspunkte. *Archiv für Begriffsgeschichte* 37: 257–284.

Sandbothe, Mike. 2001. *Pragmatische Medienphilosophie*. Weilerswist: Velbrück.
Schuermann, Eva. 2000. *Erscheinen und Wahrnehmen*. Munich: Fink.
Schuermann, Eva. 2005. Maurice Merleau-Ponty. In *Klassiker der Kunstphilosophie*, ed. Stefan Majetschak, 266–286. Munich: Beck.
Schulte, Joachim. 1990. Stilfragen. In *Chor und Gesetz*. Frankfurt am Main: Suhrkamp.
Strawson, Peter Frederick. 1970. Imagination and Perception. In *Experience and Theory*, ed. Lawrence Foster et al. Amherst: University of Massachusetts Press.
Waldenfels, Bernhard. 2000. Responsivität des Leibes. In *Merleau-Ponty und die Kulturwissenschaften*, ed. Regula Giuliani, 305–320. Munich: Fink.
Welsch, Wolfgang. 1990. *Ästhetisches Denken*. Stuttgart: Reclam.
Wittgenstein, Ludwig. 1986. *Philosophical Investigations*. Oxford: Basil Blackwell.
Wittgenstein, Ludwig. 2007. *Lectures and Conversations on Aesthetics, Psychology and Religious Belief*. Berkeley: University of California Press.

CHAPTER 6

The Constructions of Imagination

We have established thus far that seeing relates not only to things present but also to things that are absent. What is indicated here is the way imagination is involved in seeing, thereby explaining the presentational powers of the act of perception. The absence of the invisible and the imagined in seeing and in the visible presupposes "the faculty for representing an object even without its presence" (Kant 1998, p. 256). This faculty has classically been designated 'imagination.' The iconicity of seeing can be regarded as grounded in this faculty, which is, according to Kant, not only "a necessary ingredient of perception itself" (ibid., p. 239), but also the "power of representation" (Kant 2000, §17, 23, 49, 62). Arguably, it would also be possible to speak of fantasy.[1] Currently, the term 'creativity' is used in a similar way

[1] The terms are all polyvalent and their use wanders according to author, language and époch. Coleridge (1817) distinguishes between ***imagination*** as a creative faculty and *fancy*. The German term *Einbildungskraft* is translated into French as 'imagination,' meaning a *Vorstellungsvermögen*, translatable as faculty of representation. This is an important shift in meaning. The plural Phantasien (fantasies) usually signifies the content of Vorstellung, presentation or representation, while German 'Phantasie' in the singular means the faculty or power, Einbildungskraft. As Dieter Kamper (1981, p. 12) has pointed out, the term Phantasie occurs three times in the Occidental tradition: "First, as 'material' […] for dreams […] and civilisations; second, as transcendentally efficient order for knowledge; third, as the reviled minor faculty of daydreaming that mainly assumes compensatory functions." The multiplicity of the term is also manifest in the various disciplines concerned with it: psychology, psychoanalysis, philosophy, epistemology, aesthetics, mythology and, in the case of Castoriadis, political theory.

E. Schuermann, *Seeing as Practice*, Performance Philosophy,
https://doi.org/10.1007/978-3-030-14507-1_6

(Abel 2005). What is meant in all these cases is a generative faculty that explains the ability of seeing to disclose the world. The debate is not that seeing must maintain an intensive relation to the powers of representation and imagination, but rather to investigate how this relation is constituted. What we see (and hear) correlates so palpably with invisible representations that the practice of seeing can justifiably be referred to as construction, discovery and invention of self and world images. In order to illuminate this iconicity of seeing and the iconic plasticity of the visible, a concept of the image must be worked out that helps to explain the generation of images in perception as well as their expressive function. Going back to the historical discourse on imagination, to which H. Marcuse attributes the honour of "breaking through the monopoly of the real" (Marcuse 1977, p. 18), we can understand how seeing is capable of extending beyond the disclosure of facts to become an act of configuration.

Here, theory once again has to deal with the problem of distinguishing between perception and imagination. The theoretical separation is undermined in practice. A recurring pitfall for theoretical explanation is that describing the correlation between perception and presentation, sight and imagination involves separating them out, whereas in practice they are fused. The theoretical concept of practice, therefore, cannot avoid missing its mark to some extent. In theoretical description, the hybrid forms of perceptual access to the world inevitably mutate into something else. The original object resists the gravitational pull of description. Reference to 'interplay' and 'interlocking' between imagination and perception should not be understood as forgetting the insight that they are inseparable. They are instead the attempt to display the difficulties in grasping the protean interactions in between them.

1 The Powers of the Image

Seeing is proven to reside between the dimensions of *being determined* and *being able to determine*. What is seen, how it is seen and how it is overlooked are all conditioned by preformed notions and attitudes. As a result, we end up with stereotypical ways of seeing as well as the freedom to adopt other ways. The process is representational in that it is possible to develop a way of seeing that alerts us anew to the medial nature of seeing. Ways of seeing are figurative forms of mediation between the self and the world. Like a non-figurative medium, the faculty of imagination both enables and obscures relations to the self, images of the world and relations to objects. Its mode of operation is quasi metaphorical, translating one thing into another when allowing something to be seen as something else or as something other than usual. In the context of his aforementioned critique of the paradigm of correspondence, Nietzsche speaks of the faculty of imagination as "a middle sphere und mediating force [...] which cannot be left out of consideration for even a second without also leaving out human beings themselves" (Nietzsche 1999, pp. 148, 150–151), Kierkegaard makes a similar evaluation of its ability to transcend the finite: "Fantasy is, in general, the medium of infinitization" (Kierkegaard 1989, p. 60).

1.1 Spontaneity and Receptivity (Kant)

The power of imagination performs various functions in Kant's philosophical system. It is the faculty of making present what is absent to the senses, and of participating both productively and reproductively in the relation between intuitions (sense perceptions) and concepts. An elucidation of its transcendental function of the categories of the understanding is contained in the schematism chapter from the *Critique of Pure Reason*. The point of departure was the question of how concepts can be related to sense impressions. A mediation is required that can be assigned neither to sensuality nor to the understanding alone. This mediation is achieved by the faculty of imagination as the common organising principle of the two other faculties.

The faculty of imagination is the means of bestowing order on so-called sense impressions,[2] of relating intuitions to categories and synthesising them to images. Schema designates both the imaginative *manner* of production as well as its product, thus already indicating its performative character:

> Now this representation of a general procedure of the imagination for providing a concept with its image is what I call the schema for this concept. (Kant 1998, p. 273)

[2] Talk of sense impressions falls back into the traps of deliverance thinking, which the concept of schematism sets out to avoid, by making sense impressions originally inseparable from schemata.

The schema is distinguished from the image in that it is not given to the senses. It is instead the methodological prerequisite in experience for such a sensory 'given': "In fact it is not images of objects but schemata that ground our pure sensible concepts" (ibid.). A general concept can be arrived at without the immediate sighting of an object. However, for concepts to be joined to intuitions and therefore not to be "blind," they require a schema. The schema founds the coherence between sensuality and understanding. It generates patterns of regular concept building by which diversity in the perceptual world is given structure. Schema therefore designates a procedure for generating perspective and form that can justifiably be termed performative, because the procedure realises the consciousness of the object-relation.

Receptivity and spontaneity are necessarily mutually dependent. As "the faculty for representing an object even without its presence" (ibid., p. 256), the imagination transcends reality and is unavoidably productive. Yet at the same time it is determined by the sensual and is reproductive: "Now since all of our intuition is sensible, the imagination, on account of the subjective condition under which alone it can give a corresponding intuition to the concepts of understanding, belongs to sensibility; but insofar as its synthesis is still an exercise of spontaneity, which is determining and not, like sense, merely determinable, [...] the imagination is to this extent a faculty for determining the sensibility a priori" (ibid., pp. 256–257).[3]

Kant guards against the objection that his claim of a merely determinable sensibility could be a version of the myth of the given (see Sect. 1.5 in Chapter 2) by assuming that imagination is dynamic mediation. On the one hand, imagination extends beyond the sensual or precedes it. On the other hand, these precedents are sensually occasioned and conditioned. Imagination thus exhibits the same paradoxical structure that also characterises seeing. It is consequently no wonder that Kant designates imagination as an "ingredient" of sense perception, although thereby effectively excluding the possibility of a purely receptive sensuality. As conceived by Kant, representations of the object enter into perception in such a way as to render perception constitutive of the object in a way that shares features with the making of images. The initial act of perception is already inhabited, according to Kant, by a schematised pre-image, a "precursory formation" (Heidegger 1962, p. 88), as Heidegger calls it. The temporal dimension

[3]The assumption that sense is something merely determined results from this way of thinking that I have called 'deliverance thinking.'

of this image-making process is made manifest in both its anticipatory and its posterior work. In this way, perception (aisthesis) is related to artistic (aesthetic) acts of generating and coping with reality.

The imagination not only generates the unity of the manifold of sense impressions, but also the unity between self and world. It is the performative force between subjectivity and objectivity, the "binding medium" (ibid., Heidegger 1962, p. 93), as Heidegger writes, the mediating medium, in which perception and interpretation intermingle. "Without the mediating function of the imagination" writes A. Pieper, "man could, according to Kant, neither know nor enjoy. He would be divided into a sensible and an understanding creature, with no connection between them" (Pieper 1981, p. 51). Pieper demonstrates with recourse both to Kant's transcendental philosophy and to Kierkegaard's existentialist conception of imagination as a necessary condition of the possibility, as well as a sufficient condition of the reality, of relating actively to self and to the world.

In the Critique of Pure Reason, Kant's main concern is admittedly the importance of imagination to cognition. However, imagination also plays an important role in practice. Its products are relevant to practice because they do not circulate in a vacuum but are exchanged with others responsively and correspondingly in relation to perceptions and concepts. These processes of communication impose practical limits on the proliferation of imagination.

On the one hand, the prefigurations of perception by schemata also lead to conventional ways of seeing and clichés inadequate to particular cases. On the other hand, however, imagination opens potentially infinite creative possibilities. The *Schematism of the Imagination* describes the formative, constructive qualities by which consciousness develops a relation to the world. Kant's representation of this process corroborates the claim that seeing is both a responsive and a constructive act of mediation.

The risks of imagination should not be left out of the picture. Kant is well aware of the abyss harboured in the ability to infinitely reinterpret the world. Precisely for this reason, he feels obliged to stress the synthetic powers of imagination over its potential for disintegration. In his Kant lectures, Heidegger emphasised the transcendental imagination in the first edition of the critique, not only as a reason for the possibility of synthetic cognition, but also as the common root, even as the original enabling ground of the two cognitive faculties of understanding and sensuality. In the second edition of 1787, this status is removed and imagination is no longer so multiform and no longer occurs on all text levels. According to Heidegger, this is due to Kant shying away from the prospect of assigning imagination the foundational position for cognition and thus fictionalising the basis of knowledge.[4] A faculty of reason rooted in and preceded by an ulterior faculty is disempowered, endangering the rationality of our relations to objects. An unbounded, hypertrophic imagination is even more disturbing when it is accorded the systematic role of originally enabling all knowledge.

Kant's emphasis on the synthetic rather than disintegrating capacity of imagination has come under critique.[5] Yet since Kant is aware of the dangers of imagination he feels obliged to "reinterpret [it] in opposition to the insights from the critique" (Gamm 1986, p. 39). However, the matter resists this kind of exclusionary thinking. Eliane Escoubas has highlighted the extent to which imagination runs counter to Kant's architecture. Imagination is "the 'faculty' that renders the theory of faculties fundamentally questionable" (Escoubas 1990, p. 505).

2 The Images of the Faculty

The images that emerge from the performative interplay of imagination and perception are not solid givens. The intermingling of the invisible with seeing does not result in externally visible objects. Rather, the products of imagination must be regarded more as processes than as the results of construction and formation [Bildung][6] involving perception and image making [ein-bilden]. The stress is on the active character of the process; Bildung[7] means a performative activity that remains unfinished as long as seeing remains open to possibilities of seeing differently. The resulting images can still become mortified, stereotypical and clichéd, since they involve determination and exclusion. However, the important point is that

[4]Dieter Henrich (1955) rejects Heidegger's interpretation on philological grounds: Über die Einheit der Subjektivität. A reading based on the shying-theory is developed by Hans-Dieter Gondek (1990, p. 256ff.).

[5]Slavoj Žižek (1999, p. 29), for example, argues that Kant is "obsessed" with [...] the endeavour to synthesise," passing over the contrary forces of imagination, imagination as an 'activity of dissolution,' as later emphasised by Hegel.

[6]More on this can be found in D. Kamper (1998). Further readings in the same spirit are found in the collection by G. Schäfer and Ch. Wulf (1999).

[7]See the overview provided by Käte Meyer-Drawe (1999). For a more thoroughgoing account: E. Lichtenstein (1966).

such images are made possible by both perception *and* imagination and are consequently attributable neither to sensibility nor to sense alone.

2.1 Iconic Consciousness (Fichte)

Interestingly, Johann Gottlieb Fichte can be invoked as an advocate of a concept of the image as a process producing consciousness.[8] An elliptical review of this notion, leaving aside the problems of interpreting Fichte, may help to determine seeing as an action by which images are produced. In Fichte more than anywhere else, the terms 'Bildlichkeit,' 'Bildsamkeit'[9] and 'Einbildungskraft' [iconicity, image-likeness and imagination] are qualified as constitutive elements of consciousness.

In Fichte's conception, all self and world relations are generated by imagination: "We teach here that all reality [...] is solely produced through imagination" (Fichte 1889, p. 187). For Fichte, the essential character of imagination is its ability to extend into infinity. It can overstep the finite to the degree that it is free—that is, not causally determined by what is physically present. Due to its intervention, the activity of the self "must [...] extend into the unlimited, infinite, undeterminable" (ibid., p. 178). Fichte refers to the moving, non-object-like, and thus intangible, quality of imagination as flotation: "Imagination is a power which floats between determination and indetermination, between the finite and the infinite" (ibid., p. 181). It has no fixed place but rather passes between the limited and the unlimited, mediating the two.

In the various versions of his theory of science, Fichte treats imagination as the place where images are produced, developing an image theory that can justifiably be called performative, since in it images are actively produced by an I as the "performer of a performance" (Henrich 1967, p. 11). Images are consequently *modes of operation* of the imagination. We would

[8]For more on this, see W. Janke (1993).

[9]With 'Bildsamkeit,' Fichte (2000) designates an infinite capacity for further development and mutation that distinguishes humans from animals. What the human is, is not determined "but rather to all conceivable movements ad infinitum. [...] It would not be formed in any particular way but would be formable. In short, all animals are complete and finished; the human being is only intimated and projected [...] Every animal is what it is: only the human being is originally nothing at all. He must become what he is to be. [...] Formability [Bildsamkeit], as such, is the character of humanity."

entirely miss Fichte's point if we considered these processes as ever completed or final. Nor can images be regarded as reflections, copies or instruments of cognition. Instead, they signify genetic processes, movements of designing and discarding, 'deeds' of construction ['Thathandlungen' der Bildung]. As Walter Schulz writes, we need not "declare the Thathandlung a metaphysical first principle in the sense of a speculative transcendental philosophy" (Schulz 1972) in order to be able to learn something from the expression. The performative structures that Fichte describes with the term can be helpfully applied to images in perception.

The fact that seeing contains large amounts of imagination does not mean that we do not perceive the outside world. Fichte indeed emphasises seeing interspersed with imagination[10] as a basic condition of the self to world relation: "The eye [...] is the absolute first and ground of the world: Being in this form [...] is a product of seeing, produced in seeing by its negation" (Fichte 1971b, p. 100f.). The world is the product of seeing and its negation, negation in turn being due to the suggestions of the imagination and the invisible. It is in no way certain that Fichte is speaking metaphorically of the eye. With his theory of bodily being-in-the-world, the philosophy of the absolute takes its point of departure from the empirical. With Fichte, the dialectic of the visible and the invisible, fundamental to the practice of perception, can be derived from the connection between the eye and the imagination.

The images that mediate between I and world are not unreal constructions but rather are determined and determining at the same time. As J. Drechsler explains in his study of Fichte's theory of the image, "the determination of reality is the simultaneous setting of reality by the I and the determination of the I by reality" (Drechsler 1955, p. 73).

This notion would seem to open up a way out of the impasse provided by decisionist theories that offer the alternatives of radical difference or indifference between perception and imagination. As Sartre chose to do in his study on the imaginary (Sartre 2004), we could decide to accept the categorical separateness between the two but this decision must give way at some point because it would mean determining seeing consistently as sensibly determined receptivity. Alternatively, we could decide to remove the division. However, this would be difficult to justify because we would have to give up the distinction between perception and hallucination. Fichte's

[10]For further reading on this, see A. Bertinetto (2001).

philosophy of the image, on the other hand, can be read in certain texts as fictionalising the relation between self and world, though in such a way that the performative process on both sides prevents us from assuming that one side is determinative. The I is not determined by the world and nor is the world determined univocally by the I. In Fichte's understanding, iconicity is the floating mediation between the eye and the imagination. Both—the sensual and the mental—are poles between which the imagination resides.

Material pictures differ from imaginings by their place within the faculties involved in cognition. Imaginings relate to consciousness as images relate to imagination. Due to their dependence on intuition, pictures are closer to reality than imaginings. Fichte understands intuition not as outwardly directed receptivity but rather as a synthesis of outer and inner, spontaneity and receptivity. Intuition produces reality for the I. The intuition is not in opposition to the concept, as in Kant, but rather in correlation to feeling and sensibility. "Contemplation sees, but it is empty, – feeling relates to reality, but it is blind" (Fichte 1889, p. 321). Sensual and mental intuitions intermesh and become a 'looking at' with the synthetic power to unify I and not-I. "Only through [...] his own image does the I have an image of the world and reality and thence a *world-image*" (ibid., p. 22, Italics from ES). These sentences provide an explanation of what it means to say that seeing is an act of consciousness that generates images that cannot be considered representations of objects.

The notion of a sense of possibility in the world of perception is also present in Fichte: "The image of the real world is only next to the image of the possible world, next to the imagination, and is given only in and through it" (Fichte 1971c, p. 489). "The contemplation of something real as such is in no way possible except in unity with the contemplation of a faculty for making images" (ibid., p. 486f.). Imagination is the faculty for making images that is active in seeing. Its images visualise the world. After 1813, Fichte prefers to speak of 'Bildungskraft' [imaging power] as opposed to the "imagination, inclined to fancy" (Fichte 1971a).

In Fichte's conception, the main field of operation for the imagination is not in art or knowledge, as in Kant, but in the interpersonal relation between the I and the others (Hunter 1973). The I draws the Not-I-I to itself by means of imagination. "This efficacity of the two must be mutual efficacity, i.e. the expressions of both must converge at a single point: the absolute synthesis of both by the imagination" (Fichte 1971a, p. 406).

Fichte's problematic conclusion that "Pictures are [...] the only things which exist" (Fichte 1931, p. 89), could be elaborated on by adding that they are the only thing we have left in the relation to a world accessible only from particular perspectives. "Pictures which float past without there being anything past which they float; which, by means of like / similar pictures, are connected with each other: pictures without anything which is pictured in them, without significance and without aim. I myself am one of these pictures; nay, I am not even this, but merely a confused picture of the pictures" (ibid. Fichte 1931).

3 The Affective Force of Images

Kant and Fichte attribute a truly impressive power to the imagination. We cannot overestimate the extent to which it participates in all processes of world disclosure. All perceptions of self and world are inhabited by the affective power of images,[11] by an orchestral range of feelings, desires, projections and stereotypes.[12]

Perceptions of world, the self and others are influenced by images of wishes and fears, which, as we will see, in an extreme case like Don Quixote, qualify as insanity rather than perception. In general, however, the imaginary comes mixed with things sensually present.[13]

It is therefore no wonder that imagination participates dramatically in interpersonal perception. Gehlen referred to imagination as a social organ and explained its role in "identifying with another" as the "prerequisite of self experience" (Gehlen 1966, p. 318). The ability to empathise and see oneself with the eyes of others presupposes fantasy and the power of representation.

A short exemplary excursion into the psychology of interpersonal perception should make clearer the iconicity of perception from an empirical viewpoint. The psychologist R. Laing and several co-workers were able to exhibit in numerous case studies of interpersonal perception the perceptual interaction between the I and the other as an interweaving of reception and interpretation, such that perceptions acquire iconic qualities. My self-image is based on the images the others have, or seem to have, of me: "my view of the others' view of me" (Laing et al. 1966, p. 5). Consequently, the

[11] Interesting in this regard is the empirical study by James Elkins (2001).

[12] On the psychological and affective aspects of interactive percept, see the collection by Gertrud Koch (1995).

[13] See W. Iser (1991, p. 314): "The imaginary perhaps only attains to pure presence on madness."

authors speak consistently of spirals of interpersonal perception: "My field of experience is, however, filled not only by my direct view of myself (ego) and of the other (alter), but of what we shall call meta-perspectives, my view of the other' s (your, his, her, their) view of me. I may not actually be able to see myself as others see me, but I am constantly supposing them to be seeing me in particular ways, and I am constantly acting in the light of the actual or supposed attitudes, opinions, needs, and so on the other has in respect of me. From this we see that as my identity is refracted through the media of the different inflections of "the other" – singular and plural, male and female, you, he, she, they- – so my identity undergoes myriad metamorphoses or alterations, in terms of what the others become to the others. These alterations in my identity, as I become another to you, another to him, another to her, another to them, are further re-interiorized by me to become multifaceted meta-identities, or the multi-facets of the other I take myself to be for the other, the other I am in my own eyes for the other" (ibid., p. 4f.).

The psychologists designate the imaginary components of seeing as projections. But can we establish what parts of a perception are in fact projective? According to Laing, "Pure projection tells us nothing about the other" (ibid., p. 17). "This is more exacting than to assume that Peter is purely inventing his view of Paul" (ibid.). If imaginings were mere 'subjective' projections, we would be unable to explain why a particular perception is disposed to evoke a particular projection, and unable to say when a perception begins and stops being projective. Paul as he appears to Peter is the occasion of his being perceived by Peter, the 'fusion' of the seen and the figured incorporates parts of both. "Thus Paul-for-Peter is neither a total invention nor a pure perception. [..] Paul as actually experienced by Peter will be compounded of perception, interpretation and fantasy" (ibid., p. 19).

The question here is what is meant exactly by 'zusammengesetzt' ['aggregated'], 'fusion' and so on. The theoretical description of the practice as a whole repeatedly tends towards reification, in the sense of the notion of givenness. The relation between perceptive and imaginative parts is not merely additive. Without the concept that the visible relates in terms of both disposition and motivation to the act of seeing rather than causally and in a pre-determined way, we would be unable to explain what the empirical studies of interpersonal perception have shown, namely that the I perceives the other by making an image that is, as a general rule, neither mere invention nor pure replication. A faculty of imagination inherent to perception itself operates as the condition of possibility for the making of images [Bildung von Bildern] that both discover and invent [finden und erfinden] the world by more or less adequately conceiving it.

In treating the perception of self and others as iconic, perception need not imply aesthetic distance. Gernot Böhme has explained the shortcomings of such a conception: "People do not generally appear from the distance of the theatre seat and even less from the perspective of the television viewer. Touched by the air that surrounds them and spoken to by their physiognomy, they are not mere images to us, but rather the apparition of concrete persons" (Böhme 1995). To this must be added that the concrete persons also become iconic under the influence of the imaginary.

4 Corporeality and Iconicity

The systematic intent of this chapter has been to explain the iconicity of seeing with the aid of a differentiated concept of the image and its origins in the human faculty of imagination. As a picture-making creature, as *homo pictor* (Jonas 1973) and *animal symbolicum* (Cassirer 1962), the human discloses the world in a way that cannot be divided hierarchically into separate domains of competence. Attaining a mental image of an object can involve deliberately ignoring the surface, but it can also involve being blinded by the surface and overlooking what is concealed beneath it. In both cases, seeing operates at the intersection of the visible and the invisible.

The considerations up to this point have lent support from the history of philosophy to the claim that seeing is type of world disclosure. Since it is uncertain which criteria can be applied to determining this world disclosure, seeing represents one of the chief aporias in philosophy. I therefore want to restate and develop further the claim that the constellation of the viewer and the visible is a dispositional relation.

In his essay *L'Imaginaire*, Sartre asserts that perception and imagination are fundamentally separable. He must argue in this way in order to conceptualise imagination as the power to freely transcend the reality of perception. However, in the chapter on the gaze in *L'être et le néant*, this separation proves to be untenable. When Sartre's eavesdropper feels caught in the act merely by the expected, imagined gaze of the other, a faculty of imagination must undeniably be at work. If the eye were only to receive plain facts, there could be no such talk of an interpersonal visual event. The free imagination can only be defended at the price of a certain loss of reality. By the same token, seeing is reduced to a representational sense data model if the interconnectedness of perception and imagination is denied.

The formulation of this problem by Colin McGinn (McGinn 2004) also demonstrates that all carefully ordered, strict distinctions between "percepts" and "images" break down at a certain point, forcing the author to announce, against his original intention, a kind of "imaginative seeing" as a genuine form of seeing rather than as fancy [Einbilden]. McGinn wants to reserve 'imaginative seeing' for 'seeing-as' but must postulate a 'with the body kind of seeing' that he had previously eliminated as 'mindsight' (McGinn 2004, p. 35ff.).

At first sight, the obvious criteria of distinction between perceptions and imaginings (i.e. the physical absence of the imagined as opposed to the physical presence of the perceived) is insufficient because things imagined, remembered, feared—in short, things present but invisible—play into the way we see visible things.[14]

Yet there are uncontroversial differences between perceptions on the one hand, and hallucinations, illusions, fancies [Einbildungen] and phantasms on the other. Consequently, perception and imagination can justifiably be regarded as two different attitudes to content, which are distinguished from one another in terms of bodily presence and absence. Nevertheless, this does not identify an internal relation. If they develop genetically out of one another other they must be reducible to one another. After everything we have said, this is as absurd as the assumption that they are radically unconnected. As Husserl puts it, the differences between the "present object of perception and the merely re-presented object of phantasy" (Husserl 2006, p. 12), between the corporeality of seeing and the iconicity of imagination, (see Jaspers 1997) tend to collapse whenever something seen carries iconic traits and when imagination is articulated in a bodily manner, such as when Sartre's voyeur blushes at the expectation of being caught.[15] Fears and wishes can affect the body in the absence of their object. Imaginings, such as anticipation and memory are based on and can occasion somatic effects. Corporeality is consequently a material manifesting quality not only of perceptions, and iconicity is not just a quality of imagination, but rather the

[14]W. Iser (1991, p. 312) has described this concisely: "The continuity and identity of the perceived object can only be ensured by imaginary constituents."

[15]See Sect. 2 in Chapter 8. The distinction being the experience of imagining and imaginings themselves merely relocates the problem while leaving unaltered the fact of the effects of images on the body.

two intermesh in such a manner that they do not occur separately in practice. There is a problem here similar to the mind–body problem. Sensations cannot be explained either physically or mentally alone.

4.1 Perceptual Images

The relation between perceptions and images is similar to that between the ethical and the aesthetic. They are not as different as two entirely unrelated things, but they do not converge without difference either. There seem to be equally plausible reasons for their inseparability as there are for their separation. In short, it is their connectedness that presupposes their distinctness.

Seeing can be a way of constituting objects due to its imaging power, in which the conscious acts of memory, of expectation and of mental presentation are involved. Such seeing is still distinct from phantasmagoria because it is responsive. Without the concept of practice, these two aspects cannot be mediated with one another. Only the notion of practice reveals perception as a whole, in which individual acts are judged according to their intra- and inter-subjective relevance and in which there is no such thing as an original perception that can be grasped by subtracting socio-historical codes. In practice as a whole, acts of perception are ways of seeing that at the same time influence and are influenced by culture. They do not constitute an immediate relation to what is really given but are instead acts of mediation between I and world. Images develop against the background of what has been previously perceived and the perceptions themselves come about in correspondence to the criteria of images, schema and representations—that is to say, in the temporal horizon of previous experience and expectations derived from that experience. A representationalist posing of the question of how much such images can 'correspond' with their referents is answered from the point of view of performative practice not as a dual copy relation, but rather as the iterative structure of references referring to references, interpretations interpreting interpretations. This does not mean they are empty signs without a material basis. The world *is* the interpreted world. We cannot say what it would look like if it were not interpreted—that is, mediated by symbols, language and signs. Interpretations are not arbitrary constructions, but rather conditioned and regulated by the context of the practical.

4.2 Image Without Model

It would be no remarkable finding that perception is necessarily reflected, interpreted and mediated if it served only to revitalise constructivist concepts. Within a performative concept of perception, however, this result can be specified to render the mediations paradoxically both responsive and spontaneous, fictional and perceptual. Husserl's lucid qualification of the image as "perceptual figment" (Husserl 2006, p. 612) is a also just characterisation for images in perception, which then become aesthetic–aesthetic acts of mediation between self and world. Once again, the model of seeing as practice both requires and enables a break with the logic of the disjunction between subject and object, since the paradoxical structure of perceptual-fictive mediations can be grasped neither with constructivist nor with realist concepts. It lies somewhere between the two. Perceptual–fictitious mediations produce images of self, world and others that are not object-like. As problematic as the concept of mental images may be for epistemology,[16] the non-object images that someone makes of themselves and the world (see Schuermann 2005) out of perceptual and imaginary images can only be grasped as performative formations occasioned aisthetically, in which the person cannot help but undertake evaluative ways of viewing the world. Images of world and self are not only metaphors, but also the performance of perception and imagination, as iconic object relationships and non-inauthentic forms of other types of 'authentic' relation. Their authentic form is metaphoric, otherwise they would be seen to bridge unbridgeable differences between us, others and things.

If the viewer and the visible are only mediated by their performative mutual relatedness, then the perceptual image cannot be a mimetic representation. The images that generate the connection between perception and imagination are accordingly not derivative artefacts, copies that can be compared with models, but rather active processes of formulation and formation: "The concept of a picture (eikon) of facts condenses within itself the metaphysical illusion, the reversal or prejudice that phrases come after facts" (Lyotard 1988, p. 79). This illusion is purchased at the cost of an objective concept of the image. The opposition between model and copy becomes untenable if images are grasped as interminable processes of image making. The non-figurative images produced in the practice of seeing must be understood in Kantian terms as spontaneous receptivity and

[16]See Kosslyn (1980). An overview can be found in Gottschling (2003).

receptive spontaneity, as procedures of mediation by which dispositions are laid down and by which modal options are opened up. Images, as Fichte puts it, are not objective opus operatum but a specific modus operandi, a mode by which our object relations are constituted. The process of constituting an image is not the production of an artefact but an activity like 'taking in a scene' [sich ein Bild machen], 'seeing what's going on' [sich ins Bild setzen], in order to 'be in the picture, be aware of what's going on' [im Bild zu sein]. Designating images as performative acts means attributing to them a procedure of consciousness that deploys the seen and the imaginary to form object relations.

The decisive point about these image making processes [Bildungen] is performed in the interval between the self and others, between the viewer and the visible. The open process of constantly reconceiving new images occasioned by mutual rupture and reflection informs the in-between spaces[17] of performative practice in which what we hold to be real is negotiated interactively.

5 Imaginary Seeing

Image-making proceeds from seeing in the same way that narrative proceeds from doing. As we saw, it is impossible to separate perception from the insight and knowledge it occasions or mediates. What is really significant plays out between the I and the other, but also between mental representation and intuition, perception and fiction.

Undoubtedly taking in the scene [sich ein Bild machen, literally; making for oneself a picture] is an ambivalent event. Precisely because of its iconicity, seeing can miss, petrify or falsify the seen. Patterns of perception can hinder the nuanced view of things and surfaces can conceal interrelations. The prerequisite for the production of sense and meaning is the cause of both error and illusion. Images can always be both petrification and vitalisation. They open creative options of seeing differently while holding us prisoner, transcending the finite while fixing it in place. The imagination is both plenitude and void, surplus and deficit, production and destruction, gain and loss. The one cannot be had without the other.

[17] Andreas Hetzel (2004) has penetratingly described the *between*: "The performative stands for a 'between' that can be reduced neither to objective structures nor to subjective intentions. It consummates itself in our speech and action, thereby transforming or even bringing forth the subject of consummation and its framing institutions."

But precisely for this reason, iconicity of self and world relations is never entirely illusory. The mental images 'float,' in the way demonstrated by Wittgenstein for forms of life, beyond the opposition between justified and unjustified (Wittgenstein 1969, §359), true and false. They can only either remain standing within interpersonal practice, or fall if they are infelicitous in the same way Austin's speech acts.

Not every semantic seeing is a perception of possible aspects of something. There is an imagined seeing that fails within the shared perceived world like infelicitous speech acts. This can be exemplified with the help of a certain world-famous Spanish aristocrat and a no less prominent Venetian, both of whom demonstrate the opportunity and cost of a perceptual practice informed by imagination.

5.1 The Case of Don Quixote

Othello, with his talent for being blinded, and Don Quixote, with his gift for fantasy, both shed light on a type of seeing with which they disclose their respective worlds in a divergent manner, with tragic and comic results.

When Othello *sees* Desdemona's handkerchief in Bianca or Cassio's hand, he sees something *as* something else. He sees the handkerchief as proof of Desdemona's adultery. From everything we as readers have reason to believe, Desdemona's loyalty is indubitable and Othello's conviction must be a false inference. In opposition to semantic seeing-as, in Othello's case a definite distinction can be drawn between noticing that the handkerchief is not in its proper place and concluding that Desdemona has taken it. Sense perception and judgement are two precisely defined operations. In the first instance, Othello sees an object that he accurately recognises and in the second he passes from there to certain beliefs. This distinguishes his seeing from Wittgenstein's aspect-seeing.

When Alonso Quijano el Bueno, alias Don Quixote, sees windmills as giants, he undoubtedly commits an act of creative interpretation but not of possible aspect-seeing. His case exemplifies that perception maintains a constant relation to phantasm—that is, to the possible amphibolies of gaining and losing the world. Don Quixote's view leads him into error to the extent it is unconventional, innovative and productive. Art becomes madness.[18] His case can be regarded both as an art of seeing differently,

[18] On the proximity of the two, see K. Jaspers (1977).

and as insanity and loss of reality. The danger of error emerges when the individual's way of seeing departs from common consensus.

Imaginary seeing produces imaginary images based on perceptions that are not socially shared. When Othello or Don Quixote see anything whatsoever, or rather do not see it, their perceptions are generally not validated by interpersonal practice. They diverge in the manner of a private language from the perceptions around them, just as Humpty Dumpty does from conventional language use. Sancho Panza's sense impressions differ characteristically from those of Don Quixote in that his capacities of visual perception are generally restricted to conventional seeing-that. Othello's attention is deliberately lead astray by Iago. It could be concluded that the liberties of seeing-as are only arbitrary when they are not confirmed by common consensus. Practice holds them back from such arbitrariness.

These two literary heroes are such lucid examples of the connection between perception and imagination because their omniscient authors inform us that the giants are *in reality* windmills and that Desdemona is *in truth* innocent. This corrective and certainty do not reside outside of literature. Imaginings normally remain intrinsic to perception. They are often unknown to the perceiver and even more difficult to pin down intersubjectively. The audience know about Desdemona's loyalty while Othello alone, the one it concerns most, cannot, in principle, know it with certainty.[19]

There is an important difference between the two cases of blindness that must be mentioned here. Othello's sense perceptions are less foolhardy than Don Quixote's, while his inferences are all the more idiosyncratic. He diverges from his neighbours not in his perceptions but in his conclusions. Seeing Desdemona's handkerchief where it shouldn't be, is a non-illusionary perception that anyone else could share. The error of interpretation that exceeds the visible inheres in the conclusion that this must mean that Desdemona has given this lover's gift to another lover. The handkerchief itself does not demonstrate unfaithfulness. In one case, it is the imaginative or iconic part of the perception that leads to erroneous world disclosure; in the other, it is the conclusion.

The model of a division between a receptive seeing and a cognitive interpretation makes sense, not because the perception is neutral, exterior

[19]On the sceptical problem of general uncertainty, see S. Cavell (2003). According to Cavell, the piece works through the question; how can we ever know about the feelings and thoughts of others?

to concepts or innocent, but rather because Othello's convictions about Desdemona's character are more strongly based on the invisible than on the visible.

Don Quixote is a different case. It requires a lively imagination to see weapon-wielding giants in windmills. However, such figurative, imaginary conclusions are due more to aisthesis than to rational inference. If we acknowledge the interpretive capacities of seeing, we must also take seriously the way Don Quixote sees the world. There is little point in simply insisting that he is hallucinating while everyone else knows that the giants are in reality ordinary windmills. This may be true, but it fails to explain why the case is so interesting. Don Quixote's perception is interesting because it demonstrates the freedom of perception to engage in world-making and how problematic this freedom becomes when it is not confirmed by practice.

5.2 Images Hold Us Captive

Wittgenstein was right to say that we are held captive by an image (Wittgenstein 1986, §115). It is no coincidence that he makes this statement in the context of his new conception of language after the picture theory from the *Tractatus*. Linguistically, we are positively ensnared in images and narratives.[20] Every speech act re-invokes by citation things already said[21] and our perceptions are prefigured by countless images.[22]

[20]See W. Schapp (1976, chapter 4 and passim), who places more emphasise than other narrative theories on the process of self-understanding by means of language as intrication, and construes intrication in turn as practice. However, the author reduces the relation between stories and images basically to one of illustration. On this account, images have the derivative function of making the story easier to understand. They are not recognised as a proper form of story-making.

[21]See S. Krämer (2001, p. 259) on Judith Butler‘s conception of performative speech acts: "What constitiutes its performativity is not that it is an individual speech act, but rather that it evokes past speech acts in the manner of citation."

[22]Oswald Schwemmer (2007, p. 113) adopts a similar approach: "We see what we see through the images in our image-world." Schwemmer elucidates how such patterns of perception and Prägnanzprofile [significant profiles] constitute the characteristic traits of a culture in language and images. According to Schwemmer, the utopian task of art is to break up the dogmatically inclined, ingrained customs of interpretation.

The affective power of these images cannot be overestimated and their imaginary component not only opens but also closes. There is no escaping this arrangement. Creativity, on the one hand, is the condition of the possibility of world disclosure by seeing while at the same time harbouring the danger of losing the world. Analogously, the conventionality of seeing is required to sustain it in the socially shared life world while harbouring the risk of simply restating received opinion.

The examples, however, show that there is no reason to replace the notion of pure seeing with one of pure interpretation. In the nexus of perception and imagination, the one is not reducible to the other. There can be neither *mere* perception providing objective representation, nor perception providing pure invention.

The aesthetic liberties inherent in aisthetic world disclosure interact with the social practice of a given epoch. This practice conditions even the creative divergence that transgresses it. The ways of seeing are therefore never entirely arbitrary. When they succeed or miscarry, it is not because they are true or false in essence, but because they count as capable or incapable of being adopted, regardless of justification. As far as they can be said to *count*, ways of seeing are in no way arbitrary but must correspond to the dominant life form.

References

Abel, Günter (ed.). 2005. *Kreativität. XX. Deutscher Kongress für Philosophie, Vol. 2*. Berlin: Universitätsverlag der TU Berlin.

Bertinetto, Alessandro. 2001. Sehen ist Reflex des Lebens. Bild, Leben und Sehen als Grundbegriffe der transzendentalen Logik Fichtes. In *Der transzendentalphilosophische Zugang zur Wirklichkeit,* ed. Erich Fuchs et al., 269–306. *Stuttgart*-Bad Cannstatt: Frommann-Holzboog.

Böhme, Gernot. 1995. *Atmosphäre*. Frankfurt a.M.: Suhrkamp.

Bütler, Heinz. 1996. *Henri Cartier-Bresson and the Artless Art*. London: Bulfinch.

Bütler, Heinz (directed by). 2003. *Henri Cartier-Bresson-Biographie eines Blicks*. Zürich: NZZ Film.

Cassirer, Ernst. 1962. *An Essay on Man. An Introduction in the Philosophy of Human Culture*. New Haven: Yale University Press.

Cavell, Stanley. 2003. Othello and the Stake of the Other. In *Disowning Knowledge: In Seven Plays of Shakespeare*, 125–142. Cambridge: Cambridge University Press.

Coleridge, Samuel Taylor. 1817. *Biographical Sketches of My Literary Life*. New York: Kirk and Mercein.

Dieter Kamper, Dieter. 1981. *Zur Geschichte der Einbildungskraft*. Munich: Carl Hanser.

Drechsler, Julius. 1955. *Fichtes Lehre vom Bild*. Stuttgart: Kohlhammer.

Elkins, James. 2001. *Pictures and Tears*. New York: Routledge.

Escoubas, Eliane. 1990. Zur Archäologie des Bildes. In *Bildlichkeit*, ed. Volker Bohn, 502–542. Frankfurt a. M.: Suhrkamp.

Fichte, Johann Gottlieb. 1889. *Science of Knowledge*. London: Trübner.

Fichte, Johann Gottlieb. 1931. *The Vocation of Man*. Chicago: The Open Court Publishing.

Fichte, Johann Gottlieb. 1971a. *Grundriss des Eigenthümlichen der Wissenschaftslehre*. Berlin: de Gruyter.

Fichte, Johann Gottlieb. 1971b. *Einleitungsvorlesungen in die Wissenschaftslehre (1813)*. Berlin: de Gruyter.

Fichte, Johann Gottlieb. 1971c. *Thatsachen des Bewußtseins (1813)*. Berlin: de Gruyter.

Fichte, Johann Gottlieb. 2000. *Foundations of Natural Right*. Cambridge: *Cambridge* University Press.

Gamm, Gerhard. 1986. *Wahrheit als Differenz*. Frankfurt a. M.: Athenäum.

Gardner, Howard. 1989. *Dem Denken auf der Spur.* Stuttgart: Klett-Cotta.

Gehlen, Arnold. 1966. *Der Mensch*. Frankfurt: Athenäum.

Gondek, Hans-Dieter. 1990. *Angst, Einbildungskraft, Sprache*. Munich: Boer.

Gottschling, Verena. 2003. *Bilder im Geiste*. Paderborn: Mentis.

Heidegger, Martin. 1962. *Kant and the Problem of Metaphysics*. Bloomington: Indiana University Press.

Henrich, Dieter. 1955. Über die Einheit der Subjektivität. *Philosophische Rundschau* 31.1/2: 28–69.

Henrich, Dieter. 1967. *Fichtes ursprüngliche Einsicht*. Frankfurt a. M.: Klostermann.

Hetzel, Andreas. 2004. Das Rätsel des Performativen. *Philosophische Rundschau* 51.2: 132–159.

Hunter, Charles K. 1973. *Der Interpersonalitätsbeweis in Fichtes früher angewandter praktischer Philosophie*. Meisenheim am Glan: Anton Hain Verlag.

Husserl, Edmund. 2006. *Phantasy, Image Consciousness, and Memory*. Heidelberg: Springer.

Iser, Wolfgang. 1991. Das Fiktive und das Imaginäre. Frankfurt a.M.: Suhrkamp.

Janke, Wolfhard. 1993. *Vom Bild des Absoluten*. Berlin: de Gruyter.

Jaspers, Karl. 1977. *Strindberg and Van Gogh: An Attempt at a Pathographic Analysis*. Tuscon: University of Arizona Press.

Jaspers, Karl. 1997. *General Psychopathology*. Baltimore: The John Hopkins University Press.

Jonas, Hans. 1973. Homo pictor: Von der Freiheit des Bildens. In *Organismus und Freiheit*, 226–247. Göttingen: Vandenhoeck.

Kamper, Dietmar. 1998. Bild. *In Anthropologie*, ed. Gunter Gebauer, 203–213. Leipzig: Reclam.
Kant, Immanuel. 1998. *Critique of Pure Reason*. London: Cambridge: Cambridge University Press.
Kant, Immanuel. 2000. *Critique of the Power of Judgment*. Cambridge: Cambridge University Press.
Kierkegaard, Sören. 1989. *The Sickness Unto Death*. London: Penguin Classics.
Koch, Gertrud (ed.). 1995. *Auge und Affekt*. Frankfurt a.M.: Fischer.
Kosslyn, Stephen Michael. 1980. *Image and Mind*. Cambridge: Harvard University Press.
Krämer, Sybille. 2001. *Sprache, Sprechakt, Kommunikation*. Frankfurt a.M.: Suhrkamp.
Laing, Ronald et al. 1966. *Interpersonal Perception*. London: Routledge.
Lichtenstein, Ernst. 1966. Zur *Entwicklung des Bildungsbegriffs von Meister Eckhart bis Hegel*. Heidelberg: Quelle & Meyer.
Lyotard, Jean-Francois. 1988. *Phrases in Dispute*. Minneapolis: University of Minnesota Press.
Marcuse, Herbert. 1977. *Die Permanenz der Kunst*. Munich: Hanser.
McGinn, Colin. 2004. *Mindsight: Image, Dream, Meaning*. Cambridge: Harvard University Press.
Meyer-Drawe, Käte. 1999. Zum metaphorischen Gehalt von Bildung und Erziehung. *Zeitschrift für Pädagogik* 45.2: 161–175.
Nietzsche, Friedrich. 1999. On Truth and Lies in a Nonmoral Sense. In *The birth of Tragedy and Other Writings*, 139–153. Cambridge: Cambridge University Press.
Pieper, Annemarie. 1981. Einbildungskraft und Phantasie. In *Phantasie als anthropologisches Problem*, ed. Alfred Schöpf, 45–61. Würzburg: Königshausen & Neumann.
Sartre, Jean-Paul. 2004. *The Imaginary: A Phenomenological Psychology of the Imagination*. London: Routledge.
Schäfer, Gerd and Wulf, Christoph (eds.). 1999. *Bild, Bilder, Bildung*. Weinheim: Beltz.
Schapp, Wilhelm. 1976. *In Geschichten verstrickt*. Wiesbaden: Heymann.
Schulz, Walter 1972. *Philosophie in der veränderten Welt*. Pfullingen: Neske.
Schuermann, Eva. 2005. Die Bildlichkeit des Bildes. In *Bildwissenschaft zwischen Reflexion und Anwendung*, ed. Klaus Sachs-Hombach, 195–221. Köln: Halem.
Schwemmer, Oswald. 2007. Das Bild in der Bilderflut. In *Lebenswelten und Technologien*, ed. Günter Abel et al., 107–128. Berlin: Parerga.
Wittgenstein, Ludwig. 1969. *On Certainty*. Oxford: Blackwell.
Wittgenstein, Ludwig. 1986. *Philosophical Investigations*. Oxford: Basil Blackwell.
Žižek, Slavoj. 1999. *The Ticklish Subject*. London: Verso.

CHAPTER 7

Aesthetic and Ethical World Disclosure

Seeing can justly count as world disclosing if it is the performance of an act of realisation and figuration that forms images of the world by means of *both* perceptual and imagined images. The next step is to further elucidate the aesthetic and ethical character of world disclosure. We would expect to find connections between aesthetic liberties and moral conditions. The concept of world disclosure is intended to express the processual character by which the disclosed is generated according to the way its disclosure is performed rather than that it pre-exists in the manner of a substance. Criteria of adequacy are therefore lacking for the justification of perceptual images. Yet, as the previous examples have shown, aesthetic freedom as practice can be easily distinguished from arbitrary constructions.

The ethical ramifications of perceptual world disclosure are graspable in the normative and existential significance of seeing on the personal and interpersonal levels: personally, in the individual disposition to ways of seeing conditioned by habitus and world image; and interpersonally, in the meaning of being visible for the development of self and self-consciousness. We saw how the aesthetic qualities of such world disclosure are interconnected with the representational capacities of seeing. In what follows, the structure of perceptual world disclosure will be further elucidated by means of a comparison. In Chapter 5, we mentioned that seeing can justifiably be characterised as an analogue procedure disclosing particulars and similarities that elude thought when it proceeds by subsumption. It is similar in this

E. Schuermann, *Seeing as Practice*, Performance Philosophy,
https://doi.org/10.1007/978-3-030-14507-1_7

to the linguistic practice of metaphor. The following section is concerned with the internal structure of seeing as a metaphorical practice.

1 Metaphorical Seeing

We have seen that the as-structure of seeing is similar to that of the image and that a structural affinity between showing and seeing rests on this similarity. The expressive character of a form of representation is common to both. The iconic capacities of seeing constitute a mode of representation. This would seem to lead to the assumption that seeing possesses the same capacity as metaphor. Just as the metaphor deliberately transgresses rules of language to generate new types of analogy and connections, so can seeing—when it is inchoate—become the discovery and invention of new aspects of the world. We are not here concerned with the validity of seeing but want to sketch the possibilities of such world disclosure. Nor is the concern with individual, rival or compatible conceptions of the metaphor or its truth conditions but rather with providing a description of the procedure in order to contribute to our understanding of the creative potential of visual perception.

Metaphors exhibit the same as-structure as images and the seeing of images. They articulate ways of seeing by which something unusual comes into view. The possibilities of seeing that I am concerned with here consist in such ways of seeing. I am thus seeking common structural traits and parallels between iconicity, the metaphorical, and a certain type of novel or different seeing, so as to better understand the way aesthetic–aesthetic world disclosure works. In its iconicity, aspect-seeing in particular (though not exclusively) exhibits a capacity to produce contrast, which not only explains more closely how it can productively disclose world, but it also corresponds significantly to the procedure of transference, the production of similarity and of meaning in metaphor.

1.1 Transference and Bridging

Metaphors get us to see 'something *as something else,'* A as B, and thereby to "see something in a new light."[1] D. Davidson has described this as the

[1]D. Davidson (1984, p. 263): We are here not concerned with Davidson's theory of metaphor and the epistemic problems it poses. Jens Kertscher (2004) convincingly argues that Davidson's concept entails difficulties for his theory of interpretation. Samuel

main affinity[2] between metaphor and seeing-as: "Seeing as is not seeing that. Metaphor makes us see one thing *as another* by making some literal statement that inspires or prompts the insight" (Davidson 1984, p. 263). Rorty concurs with Davidson in concluding that metaphors work as "*causes* of changing beliefs and desires" (Rorty 1991, p. 163)—that is, as the cause of seeing differently. In his reading of Davidson, R. Wollheim arrives at the conclusion that metaphors turn out to be a model for the image in general (Wollheim 1991). The iconicity of metaphors suggests inversely a metaphorical quality of the image in its difference between the representation and the represented, a difference that is bridged precisely by being *conserved*. In their twofold-ness, artistic images show a certain way of seeing things. Image-seeing is in many cases a productive retracing of what the artist has previously seen metaphorically, i.e. in the idiosyncratic way she conserves contrast and difference, and then subsequently shows this in her representation. Accordingly, artistic images manifest a seeing that is presumably at work without becoming manifest when someone gains access to an unusual way of seeing.

The bridging character is one of the decisive criteria of any metaphor. It connects heterogeneous things, not least the difference between saying and showing. The type of seeing we are here concerned with proceeds metaphorically by joining different things together; it probes identity and by this makes a new image. A seeing that is creative rather than receptive performs in perception what the metaphor performs in the medium of language.

V. Aldrich describes as a visual metaphor what happens when non-identical things are seen as identical, whereby a new aspect becomes recognisable. Seeing Mary as *like* Agatha, when the two resemble each other, does not constitute seeing a new aspect. To see Mary as Agatha could be simple mistaken identity; for instance, when someone sees Mary without Agatha on the street. M must be seen as A in the consciousness of their difference for it to count as aspect-seeing (Aldrich 1996). The example shows that the notion of visual metaphor is in no way metaphorical in itself but rather expresses the powers of transference, meaning production, and demonstration inherent in seeing. We have already seen that an exclusively

C. Wheeler III (2004) positively evaluates the theories of Wittgenstein and Davidson. By contrast, Joachim Schulte (1990) is sceptical.

[2]On the comparison between the procedures of metaphor and aspect-seeing, see Marcus Hester (1966).

iconic use of verba videndi in cases in which seeing and understanding constitute an inseparable unity is comparatively rare. This is why talk of sight as insight is no pale metaphor but actually derives intrinsically from the double roots of seeing in the sensible and the mental. Additionally, it now becomes apparent that seeing in its duplicity as sensible and mental also operates metaphorically—namely when it bridges differences—thereby generating new aspects. Seeing can proceed analogically because it is capable of comparing and transferring similarities and correspondences between non-homogenous things.

1.2 *Resemblance*

According to Aristotle's classic definition, metaphors occasion perception of likeness between unlike things. Metaphors generate interconnections by suggesting contexts bound up with attitudes, practices and emotions. They thereby extend beyond the domain of propositional utterances. Aspect-seeing proceeds metaphorically when it sees something as something. Seeing what something looks like, also prompts new types of resemblance, as in the example of Cézanne. Both types of seeing contain possibilities for unfolding new, unusual ways of seeing.

With the concept of family resemblance, Wittgenstein (1986, p. 66) rehabilitates pictorial relations established by language with non-propositional expressions. If I want to explain the simultaneity of correspondence and difference under the predicates of determined concepts, the categories of identity and difference are of no help. Resemblance however is the concept that can mediate between the two. According to Wittgenstein, the resemblances between different language games employing the term game, cannot be discovered by thought but through closer inspection: "Don't think, but look!" (ibid.) Although Wittgenstein is here referring to language use and not sensible qualities, it nevertheless applies to the present case, because we need a procedure that operates differently from conceptual thought. In order to discover how resemblance occurs, we need a certain type of perception, a thinking or mental seeing directed at the *how*. Seeing-how is a non-propositional form of grasping sameness and otherness. As such, it has the same power as seeing-as to perceive new types of connection where conventional seeing only finds, predicates and appraises what it expects.

Dealing with resemblance is an aesthetic matter rather than a logical one, and it is due rather to perception than to thought. This is at the basis of the notion that "resemblance is to identity as image is to concept. A relation of identity forcibly dictates; resemblance provides connections according to the measure of the imagination" (Gamm 1992, p. 70)—that is, the imagination, referred to by Nietzsche as the drive to formulate metaphors (Nietzsche 1999, p. 150).

With reference to Paul Valéry, G. Mattenklott elucidates a concept of similarity by which it is "equidistant from imitatio naturae and from free imaginative production" (Mattenklott 2001, p. 182). Resemblance is therefore in a category of its own and is neither on the side of sense-identifying hermeneutics nor of sense-shifting deconstruction. Its power to generate style "rests at the same time on gravity and on transparency" (ibid.). With models of similarity, you avoid the pitfalls of both appropriation by classification and over-determination of alterity. Resemblance explains a type of mental operation, it is a procedure of intelligence, a balancing act of maintaining the relation to the identical and the non-identical; it is equally rooted in sameness and otherness.

If we understand seeing in this way as a balancing act by which creative connections are generated and old connections interrupted, resemblance is then no longer a property of things or their relations but rather the product of a certain way of seeing.[3] Merleau-Ponty has a similar notion: "Resemblance is the result of perception, not its mainspring" (Merleau-Ponty 1964, p. 171)[4] If this is true, then the world we see would always just be similar but never entirely identical to the world, about which we can make no statements because we can neither see it nor interpret it. "The same thing is both out there in the world and here in the heart of vision—the same or, if one prefers, a similar thing" (ibid., p. 166). This would be sufficient an argument to debunk a simple representationalist understanding of the relation between vision and the visible. Just as a perception can never quite 'do justice' to the perceptum, by the same token, the same

[3]René Magritte must have been thinking of something like this when he distinguished between resemblance and similitude, characterising his painting as a procedure for producing unusual connections between heterogeneous things. Regine Prange (2001, p. 44) explains Magritte's approach with reference to Foucault's 'The Order of Thing'' and his conception of similarity as the "Merging of thought and the world," which can also be understood as "thinking seeing or seeing thought,[...] which generates certain affinities between things that remain hidden to everyday seeing." Magritte embeds his concept of resemblance in a somewhat adventurous and unsupported theory of the "mystery." See K. Lüdeking (1996).

[4]On this point, see also C. Scherer (2001).

perception can never miss it entirely because it is in any case only an approximation proceeding more or less creatively or conventionally. The liberties of aesthetic world disclosure, which I am attempting to illuminate by means of such analogies, must hang together with such metaphorical capabilities. The picture-like character of metaphor is mirrored in the iconic character of seeing as productive world disclosure displaying the double rootedness in "gravity and transparency" just mentioned.

'Inauthentic' seeing is just as difficult to distinguish from the authentic as inauthentic speech. It is a seeing that shows something by seeing. It can show something by virtue of discovering and producing more or less unusual analogies. On account of this active character, Blumenberg and others (Strub 1991) have stressed that the metaphor belongs less to semantics than to pragmatics, less a type of statement than an activity, a 'verité à faire' (Blumenberg 2010, p. 25) consisting in displacing meaning. Metaphors do things with words by showing things. The decisive structural trait of the metaphor is its practical, active form. It "does not say anything, it does something. In other words, it does something by virtue of what it says" (Wollheim 1991, p. 30).

We can also refer to the distinction between saying and showing made by Wittgenstein in the Tractatus. Metaphors show something that cannot be said otherwise. The non-propositional aspect of their expressive power consists in an irreplaceable iconicity. In analogy to the way metaphors produce sense, seeing produces sense by virtue of a non-propositional force of demonstration. As a metaphor-like activity, seeing develops qualities of representation including the development of optical appliances capable of showing things previously unseen. As an image-making operation, perception discovers previously undisclosed states of affairs. Thus, as a mode of world disclosure, perception is all the more a form of action, a modus operandi, through which and in which we disclose the visible world that in turn presents or expresses itself to us. The meaning of the visible is many-layered. Each individual act of seeing discloses only one possible aspect and diverges from the perceptions of others not only in terms of specific blindness but also in terms of the lucidity or other features of its metaphorical capacities.

2 Normative Seeing

As the next chapter will expound in more detail, the power to see and be seen by other persons extends from acts of normative identity attribution to acknowledgement. The way people perceive the world is a form of world disclosure because it is specific to their personality, and dependent on their moral dispositions. Individual inclinations to judge and censure, to prejudice, to bias and to personal preference condition what and how we see.

Such world-images of a normative background to speech, perception and action are at once *prerequisites* and *products* of perceptive-fictive world disclosure. Instead of speaking of world-images, we could speak of the world views[5] involved in mindset, patterns of behaviour and common normative orientation. Such world-images are, in any case, evaluative presuppositions often accompanied by conflicting validity claims, and have already preconfigured vision before it is directed at the world. They are thus the conditions of possibility for creative and conventional world disclosure.

A 1930s psychological study on widespread perceptions of aversion provides an informative everyday example of the conventionality of perception and the historical variability of such conventions (Cason 1930). In the study, numerous test subjects regarded the sight of a "woman smoking a cigarette in public" (ibid., p. 187) as offensive behaviour, comparable to "[seeing] a person picking his (or her) teeth" (ibid., p. 131). This was not because smoking was seen as a health risk or the smoke seen as a nuisance, both of which apply independently of gender, but rather because it was regarded as improper behaviour for a woman, especially in public.

Admittedly, the way smoking is *regarded* in health and fitness discourses goes beyond aisthesis. However, the concrete sight of a woman smoking does not, especially when she is wearing a bob. This sight and the emotions it stirs up are very much a question of seeing, and indeed a type of seeing that is, in practice, not independent of evaluative perspectives. It is thus a seeing that cannot be performed without being a *way* of seeing.

An example closer to home with the same structure is the general acceptance, within a certain generation, of tattoos, once viewed with widespread distaste. Such normative constructions could be described as the narrative constitution of reality, since narrative framing determines how emotion-based perceptual patterns are established. Using the example of eating a cake, Charles Taylor shows how a person's eating behaviour can be embedded in totally different interpretive frameworks according to whether or not the narrator invokes cholesterol and carbohydrates or qualities of self-control and abstinence (Taylor 1985, p. 20). The salient point here is the

[5] See K. Jaspers (1994), who divided world views [Weltanschauungen] into sensible-spatial, psychic-cultural and metaphysical.

way such narratives begin with perceptions: how I literally and concretely *see* something determines my possibilities of world disclosure.

2.1 Socialisation and Social Control

An example from behavioural studies can show how social norms permeate perception. At the University of Newcastle upon Tyne, researchers performed the following experiment: "We examined the effect of an image of a pair of eyes on contributions to an honesty box used to collect money for drinks in a university coffee room" (Bateson et al. 2006). The image of the eyes was periodically replaced with an image of flowers. "People paid nearly three times as much for their drinks when eyes were displayed rather than a control image" (ibid.). Obviously, "the images made the participants automatically and unconsciously feel they were being watched" (Becker 2006). In any case, they paid significantly more often when the image of the eyes was displayed. The fact that during the two and a half months of the experiment, up to 200% more money was found in the money box at the times of the pseudo-surveillance was explained thus by the researchers: "the latent sense of being observed promoted public-minded behaviour among the participants" (ibid). The concern for their good reputation in a community was a strong motivation to co-operative and fair conduct. "This finding provides [...] evidence [...] of the importance of cues of being watched and hence reputational concerns, on human cooperative behaviour" (Bateson et al. 2006).

It was incontrovertible, even before Foucault, that being publicly visible has a normative function. That the mere feeling of being visible has a comparable effect demonstrates that the eyes exercise an extraordinary power of moral persuasion. This explains the immediacy of light metaphors in connection with the eyes. In the darkness of invisibility, we behave differently from the way in which we behave in the light of the public eye. The imagined eyes in the experiment have a similar effect to Mead's generalised and internalised other. What is interesting from the perspective of socialisation is the significant extent to which the assumption of role expectations is conditioned visually and built on the experience of being seen. Genetically, the acquisition of perceptual patterns presumably begins here.

"I am seen therefore I am;" this is how Winnicott (1999) summarises the findings from the point of view of developmental psychology. Before we can see and speak, we are seen and spoken to.

The development of sensory consciousness begins the instant the infant is reflected back to itself by its parents.[6] Lacan describes this as the mirror stage of infant development. "The child, at an age when he is for a time, however short, outdone by the chimpanzee in instrumental intelligence, can nevertheless already recognize as such his own image in a mirror" (Lacan 2004, p. 3). What I am confronted with in the mirror is not my self but rather the others in my self or the self I am for the others.

2.2 *Esse Est Percipi*

Speech act theories such as J. Butler's about the way intersubjective identity, i.e. socialisation and subjectivisation, is constituted have demonstrated the role of speech practice therein. An act of communication attributes to someone what they are or should be in the eyes of parents or other speakers endowed institutionally with authority. It seems to be all too obvious that the speech act 'It's a girl' must be preceded by an act of perception, so that this factor has been overlooked as an occurrence with a meaning of its own. But, the fact of being visible in the eyes of others has an enormous impact.

The development of self-consciousness is not a matter of disembodied speech acts but is a form of practical performance based on perceptive-fictive self images. It is here once again useful to return to Bourdieu. Whereas he initially focuses on the linguistic side of performative identity attribution (Bourdieu 1991), he later elucidates the aisthetic constitution of these processes. "The child can only discover others as such on condition that he discovers himself as a 'subject' for whom there are 'objects' whose particularity is that they can take him as their 'object.' In fact, he is continuously led to take the point of others on himself, to adopt their point of view so as to discover and evaluate in advance how he will be seen and defined by them. His being is being-perceived, condemned to be defined as it 'really' is by the perception of others" (Bourdieu 1997, p. 166).

The chances of shifting the determination made by the gaze of the other depends on a meshwork of accompanying conditions that is difficult to see through. Just as there are felicitous and infelicitous speech acts, so too can looks be affirmative or destructive. The effects of speech vary according to the speaker's institutional power and personal authority. Correspondingly, one person's look will be more powerful or violent than another's, not

[6]Also interesting is: M. Pines (1985).

least due to the influence granted them by the person looked at. To what degree an attribution *sticks* and is taken on board depends on the second person's cooperation, be it voluntary or involuntary, conscious or unconscious. Power can exercise and stabilise itself mainly because it is accepted by people because they are dependent on recognition. If, with Foucault and Butler, power is considered as a condition of one's existence, i.e., as "forming the subject as well" (Butler 1997, p. 2), then this power is not simply imposed from the outside but it must correspond to something in the subject's psyche that complements it from within.

The assumption of roles permits the practice of creative deviance. Such practices are neither entirely free nor entirely determined. The recognition of the other's power is achieved when it is internalised and the subject's embodied habitus has come to correspond to the identity accorded to them by the other.

This explains why interpersonal perception is unavoidably laden with so much affective baggage. "The whole set of *silent censures* imposed by the very logic of the domestic order as a moral order, would not be so powerful or so dramatic if they were not charged with desire and, through repression, buried in the deepest level of the body where they are recorded in the form of guilt, phobias, or, in a word, passion" (Bourdieu 1997, p. 167).

References

Aldrich, Virgil Charles. 1996. Visuelle Metapher. In *Theorie der Metapher*, ed. Anselm Haverkamp, 142–162. Darmstadt: Wissenschaftliche Buchgesellschaft.

Bateson, Melissa et al. 2006. Cues of Being Watched Enhance Cooperation in a Real-world Setting. *Biology Letters* 2.3: 412–414.

Becker, Marcus. 2006. *Scharfer Blick Augen-Plakate schrecken Egoisten ab.* Spiegel-Online, 28 June. http://www.spiegel.de/wissenschaft/mensch/0,1518,423887,00.html. Accessed 2 July 2006.

Blumenberg, Hans. 2010. *Paradigms for a Metaphorology.* New York: Cornell University Press.

Bourdieu, Pierre. 1991. *Language and Symbolic Power.* Cambridge: Polity Press.

Bourdieu, Pierre. 1997. *Pascalian Meditations.* Stanford: Stanford University Press.

Butler, Judith. 1997. *The Psychic Life of Power: Theories in Subjection.* Stanford: Stanford University Press.

Cason, Hulsey. 1930. Common Annoyances: A Psychological Study of Every-Day Aversions and Irritations. *Psychological Monograms* 40.2: 1–218.

Davidson, Donald. 1984. What Metaphors Mean. In *Inquiries into Truth and Interpretation.* Oxford: Clarendon Press.

Gamm, Gerhard. 1992. *Die Macht der Metapher: Im Labyrinth der modernen Welt.* Stuttgart: Metzler.

Hester, Marcus. 1966. Metaphor and Aspect Seeing. *Journal of Aesthetics and Art Criticism* 25: 205–212.

Jaspers, Karl. 1994. *Psychologie der Weltanschauungen.* Munich: Piper.

Kertscher, Jens. 2004. Von der Metapher zur Bildmetapher. In *Wittgenstein und die Metapher*, ed. Ulrich Arnswald, Jens Kertscher, and Matthias Kroß, 165–194. Berlin: Parerga Verlag.

Lacan, Jacques. 2004. *Écrits: A Selection.* New York: W. W. Norton & Co.

Lüdeking, Karlheinz. 1996. Die Wörter und die Bilder und die Dinge. In *René Magritte. Ausstellungskatalog*, 58–72. Munich: Prestel.

Mattenklott, Gert. 2001. Ähnlichkeit. In *Ästhetik des Ähnlichen*, ed. Gerald Funk, Gert Mattenklott, and Michael Pauen, 167–183. Frankfurt am Main: Fischer.

Merleau-Ponty, Maurice. 1964. Eye and Mind. In *The Primacy of Perception.* Evanston: Northwestern University Press.

Nietzsche, Friedrich. 1999. On Truth and Lies in a Nonmoral Sense. In *The Birth of Tragedy and Other Writings*, 139–153. Cambridge: Cambridge University Press.

Pines, Malcolm. 1985. Mirroring and Child Development. *Psychoanalytic Inquiry* 5: 149–159.

Prange, Regine. 2001. *Der Verrat der Bilder.* Freiburg: Rombach.

Rorty, Richard. 1991. *Objectivity, Relativism, and Truth.* Cambridge: *Cambridge* University Press.

Scherer, Christiane. 2001. Das Sichtbare und das Unsichtbare. In *Ästhetik des Ähnlichen*, ed. Gerald Funk, Gert Mattenklott, and Michael Pauen, 189–216. Frankfurt am Main: Fischer.

Schulte, Joachim. 1990. Metaphern und sekundäre Bedeutung. In *Chor und Gesetz*, 104–112. Frankfurt am Main: Suhrkamp.

Strub, Christian. 1991. *Kalkulierte Absurditäten.* Munich: Alber.

Taylor, Charles. 1985. What Is Agency? In *Human Agency and Language: Philosophical Papers, Vol. 1*, 15–44. Cambridge: Cambridge University Press.

Wheeler III, Samuel C. 2004. Wittgenstein mit Davidson über Metaphern. In *Wittgenstein und die Metapher*, ed. Ulrich Arnswald et al., 195–220. Berlin: Parerga Verlag.

Winnicott, Donald W. 1999. Mirror-Role of Mother and Family in Child Development. In *Playing and Reality*, 111–118. London and New York: Routledge.

Wittgenstein, Ludwig. 1986. *Philosophical Investigations.* Oxford: Basil Blackwell.

Wollheim, Richard. 1991. Die Metapher in der Malerei. In *Bilder der Philosophie*, ed. R. Heinrich & H. Vetter, 17–32. Wien: Oldenbourg.

CHAPTER 8

Seeing Each Other

> Glances, that are exchanged. This exchange […] reaches a chiasmus of two 'fates,' two points of view. […] You take my image, my figure, I'll take yours. You are not me, because you see me and I do not see myself. What I miss is the kind of ego that you see. And what you are missing, is you, the one I am seeing.[1]

What is seeing, when people see each other, when we are visible and being looked at? Human visibility is necessarily social visibility, since we are visible in a purely physiological way only for instruments, not for other people.

Humans appear to each other, display themselves, see each other. With our partly involuntary and partly chosen outer image, we show ourselves to others and offer ourselves to be perceived by them. Every self-representation is an appeal to be seen and understood in a certain way—is either mask or face [*Gesicht*]. Looking at another, taking them into view, is fundamentally different from looking at an object. The characteristic simultaneity of seeing and being seen, the dimension of appealing-to and demanding-from, the character of encounter, all make interpersonal seeing a special case of visual perception. Seeing each other remains a seeing sui generis regardless of which type of appeal objects looked at can assume and also how objectifying looks between people can be.

[1] Paul Valéry (1970).

E. Schuermann, *Seeing as Practice*, Performance Philosophy,
https://doi.org/10.1007/978-3-030-14507-1_8

The power of the gaze to constitute identity was sharply delineated by Sartre in a way which exemplifies, in ethics, what has been called instrumental seeing. Lévinas has shown how we cannot see a human face as an arbitrary object, thereby developing the ethical paradigm of self-purposive seeing. These concepts make up the frame of reference for the following elucidations.

The general structure of the way identity is constituted by social visibility can be differentiated from diverse points of view. It has aspects in socio-philosophical, psycho-philosophical, psychoanalytic, psychological, gender and power studies extending far beyond the purview of a theory of perception such as Foucault's theory of the panopticum or Lacan's notion of the gaze as object of desire. As we have seen, Butler's theory of gendered performatively generated subjectivisation and Mead's explanations of social identity constitution both belong to the broader context of seeing in relation to personal acknowledgement. Sartre's concept of the gaze—whose one-sidedness requires Lévinas' no less exaggerated counter-programme—seems to provide a better explanation of the way perception structures the social development of self. First, however, we must take several introductory points into consideration.

1 Relations of Gazing

The qualitative differences between seeing persons and seeing objects are dependent on the mutuality of seeing. The incommensurability of seeing persons and seeing objects becomes apparent in the look or the gaze [Blick], taken as reciprocal viewing and being visible.

The difference between seeing and looking cannot be determined unconditionally without arbitrariness. Following Sartre's distinction between the eyes and looking, some authors speak of the eyes as the organs of a physiological activity and looking as the socially and culturally conditioned occurrence thereof.[2] This distinction, however, merely resuscitates the traditional division of the event of seeing into visio corporalis and visio spiritualis. There can be no appeal here to the use of language. Whether I direct the eyes at something or take it into view, whether I glimpse it

[2] On Sartre's and Lacan's use of *eyes* and *gaze*, see H.-D. Gondek (1997). On the gaze as distinct from the eyes as the in-break of the invisible, see Georg Christoph Tholen (2003). Kathrin Busch (2004) speaks of the gaze as opposed to the event of the gaze to argue for a surplus of visibility analogue to that in pictures.

or look at it, makes no general categorial difference. In accordance with the approach adopted here, it would constitute a regression to misguided polarisation to assume a purely physiological, ocular activity of the eyes. A strict terminological division is therefore artificial.

A clearer distinction can be made between the gaze in the confines of human encounters and in the broader horizon of the overview or the internalised gaze that no longer needs to be present physiologically in order to be anticipated. The gaze is not only the means and medium of a communication, but rather anthropologically existential: H. Plessner locates in the gaze encountered by the other—that is, in the "elemental phenomenon of reciprocity between me and the other" (Plessner 1998, p. 180)—the eccentricity of the human, the anthropological condition that the human being can only be herself by differing from herself. "The human possesses a sense for the 'reciprocity of perspectives', i.e. he can see the other in himself, he has a sense for the mirror relation involved by virtue of his fractured selfhood" (Plessner 1982, p. 114).[3] The ability to see oneself with the eyes of another is fundamental to generating social identity: "The human being becomes what he sees himself as being. This is his freedom" (Plessner 1983, p. 116). It must be added that it is of course also the way he is determined by the gaze of others. Plessner understands human appearance not "as a mask [...] that can be removed to reveal the real but rather like the face, which conceals by revealing." The way we appear to others determines who or what we are.

There are traits of combat in this interaction. The gaze can become an instrument of domination. However, it is only in and through the gaze of the other that a self-image can develop. The self is given to itself through its visibility for others and so can just as easily lose itself in the process.

The simultaneity of seeing and being seen constitutes a self-relationship. The I differs from itself and is at once identical with itself. By contrast, the gaze of the other works like an active mirror, affecting the spatial-temporal encounter between ego and alter. Paul Valéry (1970, p. 26) writes: "As soon as gazes meet, we are no longer wholly two, and it is hard to remain alone." Yet he adds: "No matter how far we advance in our mutual perception, as

[3] In the gaze, humans develop a capacity for mimetic transformation. For this reason, the actor is for Plessner an anthropological paradigm. The actor manifests the characteristics of anthropological eccentricities like distance to self and to the roles we play, "iconic conditioning," capacity for expression, the as-structure of presentation and mental representation and so on.

much as we reflect, so much will we be different." Quoting Musil, we could add: unseparated but not united.

The gaze is a performance that founds or destroys, begins or ends something, attributing a particular form to the I gazed at while robbing it of other possible forms. It is at once a sensory and mental encounter with the power to constitute the I. Whether social conditioning and norming, repressive sanctioning or the proverbial penetrating gaze that can be felt in the back, there is no principled difference in the constitution of subjectivity. A look can move us or it can bowl us over, the gaze can be objectifying, desirous, aggressive, disinterested or menacing; it is always the medium by which an image of the self, the other and the situation is constituted.

1.1 The Look and the Face

When I look at someone's face, the eyes of the other reflect what I appear to her to be. In her expression and reactions, my subjectivity is mirrored as a seen subjectivity or is transmuted into a univalent objectivity. Hegel had good reason for criticising the missing eyes in Greek sculptures of gods as "lacking interiority," while characterising the gaze in Italian and Dutch Baroque painting as typifying modern subjectivity. When confronting the gaze in a picture or in a real face, both entail the experience of being addressed.

In both cases, a dimension emerges that we have characterised as the duplicity of seeing (re)presentations: in the restricted field of the vision of a picture, an image appears that can be different for every observer and is therefore infinite—its imaginary state performed by the viewer. Likewise, what appears in the gaze of the other cannot be frozen in time because it is at once perceptual and fictitious. Sartre understood this as the freedom of the gazing other; Lévinas, as exteriority. In both, there is something unreachable in the look of the face that transcends the face itself. This aspect is a constitutive element of the movement of seeing beyond the visible described earlier. This overreaching is a characteristic of viewing both a face and a picture.[4] In both, the visible and the invisible interplay to make something infinite appear within a finite boundary.

[4]The picture need not be a portrait and need not represent any motif at all, although representation certainly heightens the effect of address. Scenic representations of humans in action and the colour dynamics of abstract painting have the same effect.

2 Sartre's Notion of Visibility

According to Sartre, being visible means being given as an object for others and is considered to be a loss of self. The subject loses its status as subject in the gaze of the other. Being seen is the "revelation of my being-as-object for the Other" and "the presence of his being-as-subject" (Sartre 1982, p. 344) for me. Sartre here treats the gaze as the irruption of a powerful and disempowering event into the selfhood of the subject. The self loses its self-assurance and rediscovers itself in the new form attributed to it by the gazing other. The gaze has ethical weight as a power threatening the freedom of the gazed-at other. The self-consciousness Fichte was interested in becomes, for Sartre, a self-relation with a specific quality such as pride or shame.

2.1 Scopic Regimes

The other appears in my universe as the cause of cleavage and disturbance, emerging like the headlights of a police car, abruptly taking hold of me, tearing me from being-for-myself. Sartre is Cartesian enough that for him the consciousness of the other is identical with these blinding headlights: "without any defense, illuminated by the absolute light which emanates from a pure subject", (ibid., p. 384) I find myself suddenly as "a slave to the degree that my being is dependent at the center of a freedom which is not mine" (ibid., p. 358). His gaze "touches me to the heart" (ibid., p. 367).

His gaze presupposes his appearing in my field of vision, with which the possibility of the inverse objectification is always given. However, I have already lost my tranquil selfhood; the other, who takes me in his gaze, affirms or denies what I am. Being seen means self-alienation because the gaze fixes the way I am according to the way I am seen. The force of this interpersonal relation results from the fact that in every encounter I not only perceive that someone is there but also "that I am vulnerable, that I have a body which can be hurt" (ibid., p. 347).

Sartre's well-known example of someone caught in the act of eavesdropping explains the shame at the gaze that catches them in the act as "recognition of the fact that I am indeed that object which the Other is looking at and judging" (ibid., p. 350). The eavesdropper is considered here as someone who, as long as he is not caught, has no self-consciousness, immersed unthinkingly in his act. As long as he considers himself undiscovered he is completely identical with what he is doing. As soon as he hears steps and fears discovery he begins to reflect. He becomes conscious of the inappropriateness of the act and is ashamed. Here the gaze plays the role of the verdict.

Whether or not an absolutely unconscious voyeur is really conceivable, Sartre deploys the figure to bring out the process of self-becoming in the gaze of the others: "As long as we considered the for-it-self in its isolation, we were able to maintain that the unreflective consciousness cannot be inhabited by a self, […] but here [after the appearance of the other, E.S.] the self comes to haunt the unreflective consciousness" (ibid., p. 349).

Even if the steps should die away and he is not caught, the voyeur has himself become an object. The anticipated and feared gaze of the other in his own eyes makes him someone doing something improper of which he should be ashamed.

It is therefore not merely the empirically present gaze that is the necessary condition for the irruption of alterity into the being-for-himself of the subject. The assumed presence of the other can have the same effect. I can be mistaken about the presence of a danger but this is irrelevant since my self-consciousness is constituted by the internalised and merely imagined gaze of the other: "I can indeed believe that it is Annie who is coming toward me on the road and discover that it is an unknown person; the fundamental presence of Annie to me is not thereby changed" (ibid., p. 373).

This forces Sartre into a systematic difficulty. The strict distinction between imagination and perception undertaken in 1940 in *L'Imaginaire*, three years before *Being and Nothingness*, breaks down in this case. If the imagined gaze of the other suffices to bring me out of my being a subject, then it follows that the invisible and the imagined contribute to the constitution of perception. The Kantian imagination is thus an ingredient of perception that cannot be separated from it. This is precisely what Sartre seeks to exclude in *L'Imaginaire*, categorically excluding the possibility that the visible and the imagined can mix. This position is maintained in Sartre's theory of the gaze: "We cannot […] perceive and imagine simultaneously; it must be either one or the other" (ibid., p. 347).

There emerges, in seeing, a perceptible force extending beyond perception that Sartre wants to shore up with the terminological separation of eye and gaze, as it were against his own conceptual interests. He writes: "If I apprehend the look, I cease to perceive the eyes" (ibid., p. 346). As the sender of a gaze, the other is imperceptible. I can only see the eyes. Sartre thus reserves the eyes for physiological activity, and the gaze for the event with social effects. "As soon as I look in the direction of the look it disappears, and I no longer see anything but" (ibid., p. 494). Indeed, we are familiar with the experience of looking at someone else's face without realising what colour their eyes are or conversely recognising the colour of the eyes while the face vanishes. Yet it remains questionable whether the person's gaze does not remain entirely visible when I see that I am being looked at. This version is advocated by Lacan[5] against Sartre: "No. It is not true that, when I am under the gaze, when I solicit a gaze, when I obtain it, I do not see it as a gaze. Painters, above all, have grasped this gaze as such in the mask" (Lacan 1978, p. 84). According to Lacan, when I experience that I am being looked at I *see* an imagined gaze (ibid., p. 79).[6]

This disagreement in important ways resembles the one between Wollheim and Gombrich when disputing whether seeing an image as an object is simultaneous to seeing the object represented in the image. As has been argued so far, this question is less pertinent than the imaginary status of the object of seeing. Only this explains how the object of seeing fundamentally transcends the finite conditions of its appearance on the image surface or in the eyes. There are then enough arguments on both sides[7] to defend the fact that gazes can be thrown about like balls or, on the contrary, to emphasise that gazes can never be perceived and identified at the same time. However, in both cases it is the element of *overreaching* that characterises both the seeing of a face and that of an artistic image. In both there emerges an infinite imaginary under the conditions of a finite physiognomy or pictorial medium.

We must be able to see this imaginary, otherwise we would not be able to know it and report on it. In order to be able to see it, seeing must itself reach beyond the visible. As V. Descombes writes, "In order for something

[5] J. Lacan (1978). An interesting comparison between Lacan's and Sartre's theory of the gaze is undertaken by Andreas Cremonini (2004).

[6] Lacan uses the terms 'eye' and 'gaze' very differently compared with Sartre. He designates the eye as an intentional act of seeing, while the gaze is what goes beyond this act. Looking at paintings can provide "a triumph of the gaze over the eye" (109) because it shows something that is not contained within intentionality. The distinction being made is between a seeing that identifies and a libidinous desire to see that precedes it and exceeds its intentionality. Numerous newer studies are contained in Claudia Blümle and Anne von der Heiden (2005).

[7] See L. Wittgenstein (1980, 1.100.193): "When you see the eye, you see something go out from it. You see the glance of the eye."

unobservable to exist for us, we would have to be able to designate an experience in which consciousness is aware of something that presents itself to us as unobservable, an experience without which we would not know what we were referring to" (see Descombes 1981, p. 82). If the eyes only saw other eyes, we could not speak of the gaze, neither as a shaming nor an imaginary one, nor of any type of acknowledgement in the gaze. The event of seeing is literally a sensible seeing that overreaches itself by opening itself to the invisible. Without a quality of the imaginary in seeing, faces and images would be perceived in the same way as tables and chairs—that is, without twofoldness and without this overreaching or surplus.

Sartre gets entangled in contradictions typical of the myth of the given in seeing. His predicament demonstrates the importance of taking literally the supposedly metaphorical use of the term seeing and the connection of response and interpretation in seeing. Sartre needs the notion of a basic activity of the eyes in order to maintain his theory of imagination as a free faculty operating independently of physically present visible things. The imagination plays a role in his theory of seeing because the gaze is no longer attributed to "pure perception," i.e. to the activity of the eyes. As has been shown, the notion of pure perception is a naturalist reduction. When Sartre regresses to this notion, he contradicts his elucidations of the ethical ramifications of the visibility of the body. His analysis already shows, against his will, that perception is not exhausted by what is materially present and to hand. By dividing the eye and the gaze, he cannot explain the type of imaginary seeing posited by his theory of the gaze (perception under the influence of expectation and fear) and refuted by his theory of imagination, although his theory of imagination claims to offer such an explanation.

That seeing the gaze requires a concept of "imaginative seeing," as does seeing pictorial space in the exact same way, which becomes apparent when considering the intangible processuality of the gaze. Rudolf Bernet writes that the gaze is, for this reason, a "seeing with a blind spot" (Bernet 1998, p. 18). It is a relational phenomenon located *between* the self and the other, in motion between the two: "The other, who also doesn't see his gaze, is just as incapable as I am of taking possession of that gaze. We must therefore say that the gaze is located between us or *moves* between us. The gaze is thus in reality an invisible phenomenon in *transit*. Its apparition consists in motion" (ibid.).

2.2 *Acquiring and Losing Subjectivity*

As the gazing gaze, the other is not only contingently in particular cases, but fundamentally, the subject for which I am the object. The subject conceives of itself as object by grasping the other as subject for whom it is the object. This mechanical tilting is the core of Sartre's concept of interpersonality.

In the manner of the Fichtean I that can never grasp itself as I-subject but only ever as object, the I escapes itself in the gaze of the other and is evaded by the other as subject.[8] However, in contrast to Sartre, Fichte shows how an unattainable identity precedes the subject–object dichotomy, while for Sartre the whole universe exhausts itself in this dichotomy. Even God, the subject that can never become an object, is subject to his own unattainability as subject. Even he cannot "see the underside" (Sartre 1982, p. 400); he too is susceptible to the subject–object schema, because he either coincides with the totality that has no outside or the totality is the subject for the divine subject.

What is at stake in the gaze relations is freedom itself. Subjective freedom is understood in Sartre's ontology as the possibility and the necessity of choosing. I can create myself in different ways but I must create myself in *some* way, selecting from the multitude of possibilities. My possibilities are my transcendence that go beyond the possibilities of others: "the Other as a look is [...] my transcendence transcended" (ibid., p. 352). Intersubjectivity discloses itself thus as a deadly struggle for freedom: "being seen constitutes me as a defenseless being for a freedom which is not my freedom" (ibid., p. 358) and this is "the hidden death of my possibility" (ibid., p. 354). Under the Medusa-like gaze of the other, my manifold possibilities are frozen into a single petrified reality in this conception.

His freedom to pass judgement over me eludes being objectified by me. If I am at all able to refuse the verdict, to turn the tables and regain my being-for-me, it is not by perceiving the other as subject.

In the drama *Huis clos*, the servant of hell has no eyelids, so that his eyes never close and are directed continually in unbearable indiscretion at the protagonists. The famous line "l'enfer c'est les autres" speaks of the gaze as a verdict incapable of revision. If life is the openness of always possibly

[8] Describing Sartre's subject–object relation in the light of Fichte's transcendental philosophy is a fruitful enterprise. See M. Fleischer (2001). Fleischer refutes Sartre's claim that gaze relations always fail in virtue of succeeding by taking recourse to Fichte, who showed that the character of demand in the interpersonal relation of I to not-I is based on mutual limiting and acknowledgement.

being other than it is, then I am reduced after death to what was factually lived, said and done, and the others pass the final judgement on me as a coward or a hero, as the case may be. In death, the other becomes an object: "only the dead can be perpetually objects without ever becoming subjects – for to die is not to lose one's objectivity in the midst of the world; all the dead are there in the world around us. But to die is to lose all possibility of revealing oneself as subject to an Other" (ibid., p. 394).

2.3 *Master and Bondsman*

Sartre considers the relation between ego and alter as a profoundly economical, and occasionally military relation to struggle, mastery and slavery. It ends like Hegel's first stage of this struggle—that is, with the subjugation of one of the combatants. This shows up not only in Sartre's imagery and examples, such as objectifying the other as killing "the hen that lays the golden eggs" (ibid., p. 387), or the comparison to the relation between the soldier and the enemy (ibid., p. 392). It is mainly manifest, however, in the reciprocity within intersubjective hypostasis that allows no escape out of the subject–object dichotomy. The mechanism of mutual objectification is a binary either–or in which no third entity can be considered. Sartre's disjunction fends off the possibility of a successful encounter of gazes.

The one-sidedness of this line of thought has been frequently criticised. There has been talk of a phobia of the gaze (Buisine 1986), and Sartres' theory has been accorded the epithet of the magic of the evil eye (Held 1952, p. 288). His former associate Merleau-Ponty objected that "for the other to be truly the other, it does not suffice and it is not necessary that he be a scourge, the continued threat of an absolute reversal of pro and con, a judge himself elevated above all contestation, without place, without relativities, faceless like an obsession, and capable of crushing me with a glance into the dust of my world. It is necessary and it suffices that he have the power to decenter me, to oppose his centering to my own, and he can do so only because we are not two nihilations installed in two universes of the In Itself, incomparable but two entries to the same Being, each accessible to but one of us, but appearing to the other as practicable by right, because they both belong to the same Being" (Merleau-Ponty 1968, p. 82).

The participation means "that we do not have two images side by side of someone and of ourselves, but one sole image in which we are both involved" (ibid., p. 83). The other can only throw me so dramatically off centre because "we count in the same world, we belong to the same Being. But this has no meaning for man taken as a pure vision: he does indeed have the conviction of going unto the things themselves, but, surprised in the act of seeing, suddenly he becomes one of them, and there is no passage from the one view to the other. Pure seer, he becomes a thing seen through, an ontological catastrophe" (ibid).

This certainly is a far more adequate and complex view. At the same time, Sartre's exaggeration is fruitful in that it clarifies the radically interpersonal nature of perception. The systematically interesting thought that the self is constituted by its being visible for others is made clear by Sartre's one-sided approach. Self-becoming is fundamentally due to visibility and to being seen by others, such that the I of the cogito is thrown back onto its corporeality and is robbed of its autonomy. Sartre thus conceives the I radically from the point of view of the other. While remaining attached to Cartesian subject–object dualism, he breaks with the disembodied, autonomous and out-of-this-world cogito.

The radicalness of this line of thought consists in making self-consciousness always contingent upon the gaze of the other, independently of whether or not I am ashamed or proud of my act, it is always the other that gives me to myself as someone who should be ashamed or proud. Even a gaze of acknowledgement does not leave me autonomous. Being seen is always the act constituting the self interpersonally. According to Sartre, beauty, strength and spirit are not properties independently attributable to me but are instead considered as belonging to me and therefore bestowed upon me in countless looks rendering me hypostatically determined. The gaze is therefore not necessarily destructive, though always constitutive of the self and self-consciousness. Shame, fear and pride are the basic modalities of my being seen. They are the ways in which I become present to myself in the presence of the others.

In summary, Sartre's theory, partly against the spirit of its author, characterises the gaze as a performance by which and in which a shared world is disclosed perceptually *and* fictitiously. On Sartre's account, the embodying, realising dimension of effective activity renders perception an event constituting identity, making gazes comparable to acts of lingual stigmatisation and attribution. The illocutionary and perlocutionary aspects of perceptual acts are here illustrated more vividly than anywhere else. However, the one-sidedness means a concentration on the instrumental aspect of perception. Sartre's theory of the gaze shows that seeing can be used as a means of subjugating the other. The gaze appears then as a mere instrument of coercive appropriation. This is because Sartre explains seeing with the model of the ray of light falling on things previously in darkness, neglecting the systematic interconnectedness of the visible and the invisible. The typical ways of using such seeing are discovery, disclosure and judgement. In the light of the theory presented in the present book, seeing cannot be regarded as being exhausted in these functions. There must be non-instrumental forms of *seeing each other*. A reading of Lévinas can help us find these.

3 Being Visible According to Lévinas

According to Lévinas, Sartre's analyses break off too early. He agrees with Sartre that the gaze is a power that disempowers the I, but he draws different conclusions from this. By returning the gaze, the other makes it impossible to regard him as objectified. In Lévinas' interpretation, the other entirely escapes the logic of subjugation: "true exteriority is in the gaze which forbids me my conquest" (Lévinas 1987, p. 55). He conceives the gaze as a demasked and demasking revelation: "The eyes break through the mask" (Lévinas 1969, p. 66). Based on the gaze or flash of the eyes [Augen-Blick] that looks over at us from out of a face, Lévinas understands the face-to-face encounter as living epiphany.

3.1 *Face-to-Face and Alterity*

In the figure of the face-to-face, the irreducible alterity of the other is revealed. Lévinas indicates: "The way in which the other presents himself, exceeding the *idea of the other in me*, we here name face" (Lévinas 1969, p. 50). The face is thus not first and foremost a phenomenon, especially not in the sense of a piece of physiognomy, but rather a movement of transgression. The transgression takes place at the limit between the visible and the invisible. The face is more than visible. As a phenomenon that is "a certain non-phenomenon" (Derrida 2001), the other is too moved and enigmatic to be objectified. It is at once gaze and address. As address, it voices its demand, which can only be addressed in turn in the vocative, not objectified in the accusative.

The other enters my field of vision as something that befalls me. In Rudolf Bernet's description, as a circular movement: "the apparition of the other comes from the other and returns to the other after having changed everything on its way" (Bernet 1998, p. 20).

By virtue of the irreducible alterity that the face reveals, the relation between self and other is, for Lévinas, asymmetric. The other holds me captive with the nakedness of his face. From his face, he looks at me with his vulnerability and mortality, binding me to an unconditionally ethical responsibility. I cannot see at all without being committed in this way. The face emanates an imperative that I cannot evade. The nakedness of the face of the other resists appropriation and objectification. Seeing the face means experiencing something unreachable and irreducible. The sight discloses the experience of the interiority of the other, which is the power by which the other resists appropriation: "By virtue of the dimension of interiority each being declines the concept and withstands totalization" (Lévinas 1969, p. 57). What appears here as the horizon is positive infinity. "The Other remains infinitely transcendent, infinitely foreign" (Lévinas 1969, p. 194). The face opens something that at the same time overreaches sensibility, breaking out of the form it is framed within. The face does not "signify" anything; it is itself the image of God.[9]

The other looks at me from "the total nudity of his defenceless eyes" (Lévinas 1969, p. 199), and it is his defencelessness with which he guards against attack. Because he is unprotected, he is protected against appropriation so long as I hear his appeal, and when I cease to do so, I do not thereby invalidate the principle. The principle means that even the refusal to hear the appeal is an answer to it. I must in any case answer the undeniable call to unconditional responsibility. "The I is unique in that no-one can respond in my stead. Before the other, the I is infinitely responsible" (Lévinas 1999, p. 224f.). In this way, the absolute moral responsibility involved in the face-to-face 'appears' a paradox comparable to Kant's fact of reason. Lévinas qualifies intersubjectivity as the "the first event of the encounter" (Lévinas 1969, p. 199), which has nothing more to do with intentionality. "To encounter another person means to be kept awake by an enigma" (Lévinas 1999, p. 120). It is an encounter without the characteristics of knowledge. Knowledge postulates something as something, disregarding, according to Lévinas, the alterity and singularity of the particular. Knowledge mirrors and recognises only itself, never the radically alien. The face, however, "disorients the intentionality that sights it" (Lévinas 2003, p. 33).

[9]As Derrida (2001) observes, the notion of the image of God may render the concept of the face metaphorical: "conceived on the basis of a doctrine of analogy, of 'resemblance,' the expression 'human face' is no longer, at bottom, as foreign to metaphor as Levinas seems to wish."

3.2 *Non-sensory Seeing*

Lévinas and Sartre agree in considering seeing violence. Lévinas' critique of oculocentrism is directed against the Western hegemony of the eye as the organ of a perspectival striving for domination. According to this interpretation, seeing serves knowledge and its claim to power. It is a classificatory identification of what is revealed to the light of reason and stands in the violent tradition of what Lévinas criticises as the metaphysics of presence and light. Light itself he regards as a metaphor of power, the accomplice of predicative and totalising reason, whose logic is a thinking of identity that excludes alterity. The light of reason is the same as Sartre's headlights, making the other visible only as object. In Lévinas' critique of metaphysics, seeing is generally panoramic and blind to singularity, and the visible appears as the violent exclusion of the invisible. Lévinas sees this mechanism as having been at work since Plato.[10] Western reason is fixedly aimed at recognising, understanding and taking possession. As Derrida explains, "to see and to know, to have and to will, unfold only within the oppressive and luminous identity of the same; and they remain, for Levinas, fundamental categories of phenomenology and ontology" (Derrida 2001, p. 114). Lévinas trusts the word and language more than the senses.[11] To listen to the word is more significant for him than to see an idea. The biblical ban on images is easy to recognise here and the core phrase of Jewish belief "hear O Israel!" (Deuteronomy 6:4). With the conceptual figure of the face, Lévinas attempts to free seeing from the character of a verdict which it has in Sartre. The price of this, however, is the loss of sensibility in seeing: the epiphany of seeing the face is "a relationship different from that which characterizes all our sensible experience" (Lévinas 1969, p. 187). This separation is marked by quotation marks. "Vision" refers to another modality of experience, "a 'vision' without image, bereft of the synoptic and totalizing objectifying virtues of vision; a relation or an intentionality of a wholly different type" (Lévinas 1969, p. 23), that rather has the character of a tender

[10] There is one significant exception to this: the Platonic idea of the Good as beyond essence, with an exception: Επεκεινα της ουσιας (Platon 2003, 509b). It is apparent which elements of the tradition his critique of metaphysics neglect and which are emphasised.

[11] Lévinas (1991) is consistent in turning away from seeing entirely and instead focuses on a phenomenon that is no longer visual. In his late work, the figure of the face recedes and is replaced by speech. In the very performance of speaking that precedes all particular things spoken, I become meaningful for the other and expose myself as someone woundable to the other's potential attacks.

caress. There is a certain affinity here between Lévinas and Merleau-Ponty, who understands seeing as a chiasm between touching and being touched. For Merleau-Ponty, seeing appears even within its performance as passive and affected by the happening, which actively addresses the other in the midst of the passivity of its being seen. Touching is conceived as a quality of being touched.

The touch is admittedly as ambivalent[12] as seeing, since it is at once sensible and non-sensible: "The caress, like contact, is sensibility. But the caress transcends the sensible. The caress consists in seizing upon nothing, in soliciting what ceaselessly escapes its form toward a future never future enough, in soliciting what slips away as though it were not yet. It searches, it forages. It is not an intentionality of disclosure but of search: a movement unto the invisible" (Lévinas 1969, p. 257f.). Lévinas attempts in this way to conceive a seeing that is closer to an encounter than to knowledge.

The same applies to the concept of the trace. The trace is the visible absence of the invisible, breaking with the primacy of presence. Lévinas sees in the concept of presence the violent exclusion since Parmenidean ontology of non-being and non-beings out of the totality of the identical, the degradation of the absent and the negative. The trace, however, makes it possible to conceive presence and absence, visible and invisible, as intertwined. The Other is not actually given but rather absent-present in the trace. The trace of the Other is a residue of the past but also announces the absence of the future, thereby paradoxically eliminating linear time. In becoming aware of the face, we go after the trace of the invisible.

Here the motif of the commonality between seeing faces and seeing images recurs. Infinity is seen within the finite, an imaginary element in physiognomy, something immaterial in artistic material.

4 Re-visions

Whereas Sartre sees the I as objectified by the other, the seeing I in Lévinas is affected by an exteriority of the other I cannot assimilate. In Sartre, the other looks at me with a powerful "evil eye." In Lévinas, the speaking face imperatively summons me to a responsibility I cannot rescind. Where Sartre speaks of subjugation, Lévinas speaks of responsibility. Sartre's other is the unconditional power that will disempower me unless I disempower

[12] On the problem of touch, see Erwin Strauss' (1956) distinction between gnostic and pathetic touch. Also Bernhard Waldenfels'(1995) elucidations; and Antje Kapust (1999).

it first. Lévinas' Other is the unconditional alterity that disempowers me if I attempt to gain power over it.

What is common to both philosophers is that they derive the constitution of the self from its being looked at by the other. In both cases, the performance of vision is the foundation of intersubjective reality. In both there is a fundamental surplus involved in seeing between persons that extends beyond the visibility of the physiognomy. Both results contribute to a philosophy of perception by illustrating the practical character of interpersonal seeing and visibility, and its meaning as ethical world disclosure.

If we are tempted to object with Wittgenstein—'But that is not seeing!'—we must at the same time enjoin, again with Wittgenstein—'It certainly is seeing'—since it shows that social visibility is based on being visible in a physiological sense and being seen as the subject of perceptual and fictitious gazes. The separation of physiological and social visibility hence proves to be as untenable as the distinction between the eye and the gaze or between 'pure seeing' and its interpretation. Blushing with shame or turning pale with anger can hardly be seen as 'purely physiological' reactions. Instead, psychic dispositions manifest physiologically, otherwise we would not be aware of them. Indeed, as reductionist as the assumption of purely physiological seeing is, the notion that people can be visible in a purely physiological sense is just as unacceptable. We have seen how both philosophers, despite their insights, tend toward dividing and ranking acts of the consciousness participating in seeing, thereby falling back into the subject–object dichotomy. This entraps them inevitably in all the difficulties evaded by a concept of seeing as practice. They separate sensibility and meaning, construction and response, and take only one side of the two poles between which seeing takes place. With the terminological distinction between the eye and the gaze, Sartre attempts to separate receptivity from the freedom of seeing, renewing the old binary oppositions and entangling himself in contradiction. Furthermore, given his adherence to Cartesian premises, he must exclude the possibility of successful acts of seeing and the intersubjective relations beyond economy and domination. For his part, Lévinas attempts to subvert the kind of identificatory thinking and instrumental seeing described by Sartre, but at the price of depriving perception of its sensible aspect. He emphasises seeing as the awareness of an apparition without appropriating or assimilating it, but he does this by putting seeing in quotation marks instead of understanding it as a sensible, physical act. There is also reason to doubt that Lévinas' emphasis on the disempowering I is strictly a reversal of the logic of identity he is critiquing. Instead of the self assimilating the other, I am taken hostage by the other. Both theories are therefore a regression from Merleau-Ponty's conception of the gaze as interlacing, in which the active and the receptive are always united. In Merleau-Ponty, the logical structure of reversibility assumes the place of Sartre's dichotomy and Lévinas' asymmetry, and is therefore a more just representation of the ambiguity of seeing than is subject-object thinking and object-subject thinking.

References

Bertnet, Rudolf. 1998. Das Phänomen und das Unsichtbare. *Internationale Zeitschrift für Philosophie* 1: 15–30.

Buisine, Alain. 1986. *Laideur de Sartre*. Lille: Presses Universitaires de Lille.

Busch, Kathrin. 2004. *Geschicktes Geben*. Munich: Fink.

Cremonini, Andreas. 2004. *Die Durchquerung des Cogito*. Munic: Fink.

Derrida, Jacques. 2001. *Writing and Difference*. London: Routledge.

Descombes, V. 1981. *Das Selbe und das Andere*. Frankfurt am Main: Suhrkamp.

Fleischer, Margot. 2001. Das ursprüngliche Verhältnis zum Anderen bei Sartre ("Der Blick") und die unverzichtbare Gegenposition Fichtes. In *Transzendenz und Existenz*, ed. Manfred Baum and Klaus Hammacher, 61–100. Amsterdam: Editions Rodopi.

Gondek, Hans-Dieter. 1997. Der Blick zwischen Sartre und Lacan. *RISS* 37/38: 175–196.

Held, René. 1952. Psychopathologie du regard. In *L'évolution psychiatrique*, April/June, 222–254.

Kapust, Antje. 1999. *Berührung ohne Berührung*. Munich: Fink.

Lacan, Jacques. 1978. Of the Gaze as Objet Petit a. In *The Seminar of Jacques Lacan: The Four Fundamental Concepts of Psychoanalysis*, Book 11, 67–119. New York: Norton.

Lévinas, Emmanuel. 1969. *Totality and Infinity*. Pittsburgh: Duquesne University Press.

Lévinas, Emmanuel. 1987. *Collected Philosophical Papers*. Dordrecht: Springer.

Lévinas, Emmanuel. 1991. *Otherwise Than Being or Beyond Essence*. Dordrecht: Kluwer.

Lévinas, Emmanuel. 1999. *Die Spur des Anderen*. Freiburg: Alber.

Lévinas, Emmanuel. 2003. Signification and Sense. In *Humanism of the Other*. Champaign: University of Illinois Press.

Merleau-Ponty, Maurice. 1968. *The Visible and the Invisible*. Evanston: Northwestern University Press.

Platon. 2003. *Platonis Respublica*. Oxford: Oxford University Press.

Plessner, Helmuth. 1982. Trieb und Leidenschaft. In *Mit anderen Augen*, 110–123. Stuttgart: Reclam.
Plessner, Helmuth. 1983. Über Menschenverachtung. In *Gesammelte Schriften, Vol. VIII*, 105–116. Frankfurt am Main: Suhrkamp.
Plessner, Helmuth. 1998. Zur Anthropologie der Nachahmung. In *Anthropologie*, ed. Gunter Gebauer, 176–184. Leipzig: Reclam.
Sartre, Jean-Paul. 1982. The Look. In *Being and Nothingness*, 340–400. New York: Washington Square Press.
Strauss, Erwin. 1956. *Vom Sinn der Sinne*. Berlin: Springer.
Tholen, Georg Christoph. 2003. *Die Zäsur der Medien*. Frankfurt am Main: Fischer.
Valéry, Paul. 1970. Odds and Ends. In *The Collected Works of Paul Valéry, Vol. 14*, 1–156. Princeton: Princeton University Press.
Von der Heiden, Anne et al. (eds.). 2005. *Blickzähmung und Augentäuschung*. Berlin: Diaphanes.
Waldenfels, Bernhard. 1995. Verflechtung und Trennung. In *Deutsch-Französische Gedankengänge*, 346–382. Frankfurt am Main: Suhrkamp.
Wittgenstein, Ludwig. 1980. *Remarks on the Philosophy of Psychology, Vol. 1*. Oxford: Blackwell.

CHAPTER 9

Seeing Art

The free field of aesthetic experience provides a suitable illustration for the world-disclosing power of seeing. Consequently, this last chapter is the attempt to enter into dialogue with visual art. In experiencing of art works, the viewer is confronted with visual artefacts the reflexive and performative character of which makes them illustrations of processes of perceptual world disclosure. The type of seeing that is reflected through art is especially fruitful for a theoretical consideration of perception because the artist's gaze and work moulds the visible world into a point of view that breaks with those habits of seeing aimed at confirming prior knowledge and control. In art, as a means of interrupting socially authorised routines of perception, seeing transcends its denotational function to become a methodical practice of seeing differently and seeing difference.

The reality of artistic experience can only be articulated at the cost of being conceptualised, and seeing itself is something other than seeing adapted to speech. Practice is once again unavoidably foiled by theory. Philosopher C. Menke has described this dilemma: "The aesthetic experience can only be expressed in interpretive speech by suspending the impression of the adequate rendition of the properties of the object of the experience, an impression that is constituted by the continuity between propositions. The basis of aesthetic interpretation is for this reason an inseparable unity of blindness and insight" (Menke 1991, p. 135). In what follows, we will be concerned both structurally and semantically with this interplay

E. Schuermann, *Seeing as Practice*, Performance Philosophy,
https://doi.org/10.1007/978-3-030-14507-1_9

between blindness and insight. Structurally, such interlocking is unavoidable, but it is at the same time instructive semantically, in helping to explain the relation between the visible and the invisible as a relation between figure and ground.[1]

1 The Art of Seeing Differently and Seeing Difference

Just as narrative speech becomes a more or less artful act of configuration, so does seeing become an art of seeing differently by breaking with prevalent habits of seeing and by making images. Visual arts are thus a perceptual procedure of breaking with the habits of the sense of sight and of penetrating beneath the surfaces of things. This kind of approach to reality could be regarded as a mode of experience in which the usual rules are violated—that is, as the opposite extreme of conventional seeing. H. Plessner has described a method for this type of fresh seeing as the precondition for any understanding of the world: "You have to have been unfaithful to the zone of familiarity in order to see it again, [...] the art of the estranged gaze thus fulfils a necessary requirement of all real understanding" (Plessner 1982, p. 169). Genetically, the ability to see differently invoked by Plessner often develops out of pain, out of the experience of suffering, of fright and alienation; "pain as the eye of the mind." This seeing "with other eyes" establishes connections between otherwise unconnected entities, transfers familiarity to strange things, producing images by interpreting, configuring, imagining, injecting itself and inventing. Paul Valéry called this the "gift of the weird gaze" (Valéry 1970). What Nietzsche referred to as an "aesthetic relation" can be understood as a unique kind of seeing that does not subjugate itself to concepts, does not subsume the richness of sensory intuition under the Kantian schema, does not engage in "the construction of a pyramidal order based on castes [sic] and degrees," nor a "world of laws, privileges, subordinations, definitions of borders" (Nietzsche 1999, p. 146), but rather liquefies coagulated metaphors and clichés.

[1] Interestingly, Jacques Rancière (2007, p. 13) qualifies the rupture between classical and modern art as the difference in the way they relate the visible and the utterable to the invisible and non-representable. This consists in the fact that words and forms, the sayable and the visible, the visible and the invisible, are related to one another in accordance with new procedures."

When understanding is perplexed and expectations are foiled, things appear to be different from usual. We recognise here a systematic procedure of both art and philosophy. Both endeavour to envisage states of affairs other than is customary, from other perspectives, thereby robbing the conventional expectations of their self-evidence.

1.1 Image and Gaze

We now turn from the art of the estranged gaze once again to the structural moment of social visibility. As we have seen, the gaze is the point of comparison between seeing one another and seeing representations. In both cases, there is a process in which the sensible goes beyond itself within itself. As an enigmatic expression appears in someone's physiognomy, so too does an imaginary occurrence appear in the material medium of an artistic representation that can be interpreted in infinitely/many different ways (see Gamm and Schuermann 2007). Images and gazes have in common that they both provide a view that addresses the viewer in such a way that she cannot remain anonymous and concealed. The image is what the gaze hits upon, but also what forms the gaze[2] and responds to it. James Elkins describes the phenomenon using the example of Rembrandt's faces: "The object stares back" (Elkins 1996). G. Didi-Huberman put it succinctly, "ce que nous voyons, ce qui nous regarde" [what sees us, what we look at].[3]

The question of the gaze of the artwork suggests portrait painting and photography. We turn instead to a video installation by Gary Hill. The medium of the moving image, in which, for example, the eyes are blinking, produces suggestive experiences of the gaze. Rembrandt is reported to have said he paints portraits and nothing else since his genre and historical paintings *portray* the motif individually. If we observe how convincingly works express the character of their objects, every great artwork will probably prove to possess the function of memorial and the actualising force of presence inherent in portraiture.[4] The following analyses are intended

[2]Georges Salles (2001), the former conservator of the oriental antique collection at the Louvre, has given penetrating elucidations of this.

[3]With the French *regarder*, Didi-Huberman (1992) intends the two meanings the word also has in English: *to look* and, in the reflective form, *to concern*.

[4]See Jean Luc Nancy (2000), who distinguishes three different functions of the portrait: ressembler, rappeller and regarder: resemble, remind, regard, respectively.

strictly as examples. Since we are not proceeding historically, the aim is to illustrate the object of investigation using somewhat arbitrary examples.

2 Gary Hill: The Power of the Gaze

The work "Viewer" (1996) by the American video artist Gary Hill (Fig. 1) shows 17 life-sized people against a black background. Almost motionless, the figures look back at the viewer. Middle-aged men from different ethnic backgrounds look out of the projection. Their everyday clothes and their non-professional comportment have the appearance of the incidental, as though Hill had placed them before the camera without any further dramatic instructions. The casualness is clearly part of the programme by means of which the artist deliberately pursues specific aims. The people shown occasionally appear uneasy and this feeling is transferred to the viewer, who in turn begins to lose his status as mere observer. Hill's work consists in organising this confrontation between the observed and the

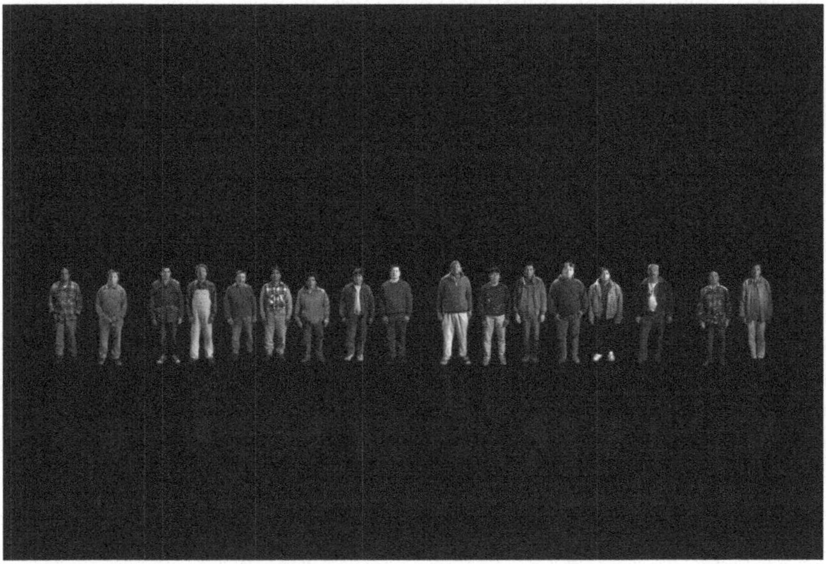

Fig. 1 Gary Hill, *Viewer*, 1996, five-channel video installation, Install 1 (*Source* © VG Bild-Kunst, Bonn 2018)

observers. Experiencing the work means undergoing the unsettling situation of looking at people looking. The shots are synchronised to put the people in a continuous row although they have been filmed separately. Slight movements occur occasionally, such as shuffling from one foot to the other, but there is no interaction. The realistic effect of being on the same level as the people looking at us contributes to the significance of the gazes.

Asked about the work's genesis, the artist explained that he invited unemployed day labourers and Mexican immigrants into his studio. However, he meant "day laborers not as a statement," but was concerned with "the notion of the Other" (Hill 1999, p. 72). The confrontation with the other in its penetrating alienness is indeed a dominant impression from the work.[5]

The situation quickly develops the peculiar character of interrogation: "Who do you think you are?" The observer sees herself surrounded by people who form a barrier of gazes, being looked at and looking at one another. Who is looking at whom? Who are these people? What are we doing here? In seeing, we appear to one another as images and are ignorant of who or what the other is. If you are disturbed by the phenomenon, you look more closely. The work situates the observer in the midst of an experience of seeing, as well as in one of apparent being-seen. The figures in the image, assuming they can be referred to as such, are observers, just as, inversely, every observer has to feel like an observed image. The fact that the viewers are in the majority heightens the sense of encounter. At the same time, any attempt at encounter seems doomed to fail since the viewers look out of the image into Hill's camera with the indifferent eyes of just such a camera. The gaze hits the exterior surface, suppressing the interior. The visible obstructs an invisible.

The theoretical considerations of seeing re-emerge in the artwork as the sensible experience of the perplexities of social visibility and thus literally acquire manifest intelligibility. The work is able to let things be experienced as enigmas—that is, they appear in their openness as indeterminable.

Hill's video installation makes manifest exemplarily that seeing need not consist in determining the visible, in fixing its identity, but can be, rather, the awareness of something, the otherness of which is fundamentally

[5]The many close-circuit Video works from the 1970s were about confronting the self as the other. Hill's piece is about the self *of* the other, who we are supposed to bear seeing.

indeterminable. What makes the viewers so unsettled is an alienness that makes them resist being grasped as objects.

What thereby becomes tangible to experience is not only the uneasiness and indiscrete power of the gaze but also the self-purposive nature of an act of seeing that is not exhausted in taking in the other but also includes withstanding his inaccessibility.

Because our attention is directed both at the representation and the represented, we understand that seeing and being visible are treated here in diverse ways: as the object of the artwork, and also as the mode of its realisation in the aesthetic experience. The experience constitutes the performative link between the configuration of the work and the power of reformulation inherent in seeing. The experience is what *puts the work on stage*, in a manner of speaking, a work whose content and form, to put it in classical terms, are seeing itself.

Traditional painting depicts figures looking out of the image in order to manifest the fact of representation.[6] Hill's case is a particularly acute version of the theme due to the specifically performative power of articulation in the medium of video. In order to test this assertion, using other examples, we now investigate the character of address and demand in the gazing image. Several examples from the oeuvre of Rembrandt provide a pre-emptive response to the objection that the suggestive force of Hill's work is primarily due to the hyperrealism of the medium of video projection and that a more self-evidently fictional gaze would be less effective in creating the impression of being seen.[7]

2.1 Rembrandt 1: The Status of the Image

Rembrandt's painting 'Susanna at the Bath' (Fig. 2) was painted in 1647. Numerous preparatory studies and drawings evince the artist's intensive

[6] Alfred Neumeyer (1964) explained in this vein the gaze, framing and internal divisions in images as aesthetic measures for removing borders.

[7] For the aspect of the imaginary that opens up the image and co-performs iconic seeing, it would be worthwhile considering the gazes out of the image in Rembrandt's group portrait "De Staalmeesters" where the gazes are not directed at the observer but, as in Velasquez' "Las Meninas," at a space in front of the space seen in the painting. Max Imdahl (1996) analysed this phenomenon. In the present book, the concern is more with the gaze as a form of communication between the image and the observer.

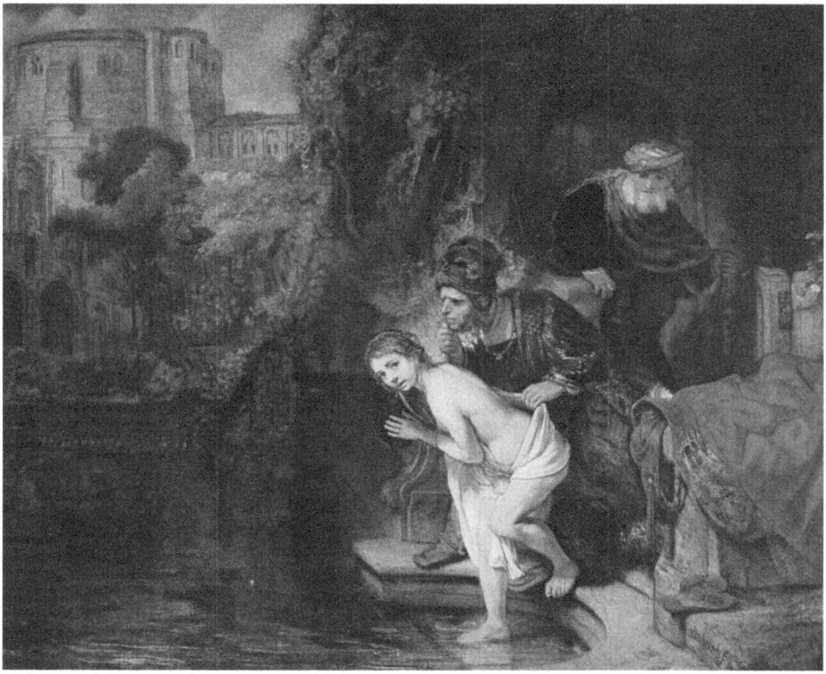

Fig. 2 Rembrandt Harmenszoon van Rijn, *Susanna and the Elders*, 1647, Gemäldegalerie Berlin

work on the motif.[8] According to an apocryphal text from the Book of Daniel, Susanna is surprised at her bath by two men and blackmailed. Either she submits to their desires or they will defame her by accusing her of adultery. She has the dilemma of either factually committing adultery before God or seeming to commit adultery before the people. The prophet will later solve the problem by causing the men to be found guilty of lying. In the moment depicted in Rembrandt's painting she cannot know this and must decide.

Rembrandt's coup consists in resolving the heroine's plight by having her look out of the image in a focused, appellative, confrontation. This

[8]On Rembrandt's treatment of the theme, see M. Bockemühl (1985).

measure decisively alters the representation. The scene becomes a question on the status of the image. The image and the viewer exchange roles. The invisibility of the observer is negated. Because the figure looks to the observer, the observer cannot appraise her while remaining uninvolved but is themselves addressed by her eyes. The image ceases to be a transparent surface permeated by the gaze of the observer to a back layer, the visibility of which is not reflexively manifested. The figure appears to know she is being seen. This is a rupture with the finestra aperta[9] paradigm of earlier painting. The image space opens into the real space occupied by the viewer, instead of being the framed view of a hermetically sealed whole with its own perspective. The gaze out of the image bridges the difference between the view shown and the viewer, creating an experiential continuum between deixis and aisthesis. This gaze opens up the aesthetic barrier[10] for communicative exchange between the realities inside and outside the image. The barrier is the precondition of both severance and meeting. Images that do not establish such an exchange of looks remain, by virtue of their frames, closed in on themselves and bordered off from the outside. By contrast, the gaze cast out of the image transgresses the frame. As Simmel writes in his *Versuch über den Bildrahmen* [Essay on the Picture Frame], the aesthetic border becomes a "locus of continuous exosmosis und endosmosis" (Simmel 1995b, p. 101).

As a result, the object represented becomes oddly opaque, akin to a window glass deprived of transparency by light reflections, throwing the gaze back instead of letting it pass to the space behind. The image thereby undergoes a change of aspect. In the categories borrowed by Michael Fried from eighteenth century French painting, the representation alters its theatrical character because the figures represented seem not to be absorbed by what they do and what they are (Fried 1980). Susanna evades absorption from the scene represented by switching over to the level of representation.

2.2 Fictitious and Imagined Gazes

It has become sufficiently evident that the gaze out of the image does not require the realism of video in order to stage the power of the gaze. For the

[9]See L. B. Alberti (1970). An illuminating commentary on the consequences of this model of the image and of seeing is found in: Joel Snyder (2002).

[10]For more on this concept, see G. Boehm (1973).

dialogical character of address and demand in the exchange of gazes, the painted gaze is just as convincing. The medium-specific effect of Hill's work consists in the motion of the video projection that is particularly well suited to illustrating the performativity of seeing. Hill renders seeing itself vividly clear as a self-purposive activity that does not lead to any determination of who or what is being seen. The entire context of the installation hinders any seeing of the men displayed as objects. Instead, we find ourselves in the midst of an event characterised by the effects of amphibolic reversal between viewing and being visible. The medium of the video projection is well-adapted to this particular form of perception and appearance. The minimal yet lively movement of the images in which the figures express their unease is fundamental to the authenticity of the inquiry undertaken in Hill's piece.

Yet from the point of view of the question of the gaze, there is another matter of more interest than the specifics of the medium. The knowledge that the gazes we are seeing are fictitious, whether painted or filmed, in no way cancels out the impression of being addressed. In Hill and Rembrandt, the imagined gazes generate as much exchange as intersubjective gazes. There is the same presence of the invisible in the visible—i.e. of the imagined, anticipated, hypothetical and so on—that is also there when we look at other people. The sense of Sartre's voyeur that Anny is approaching opens its own border within the image but in the reverse direction. The imagined gaze from Sartre's eavesdropper extends from the real situation into the imaginary. Inversely, the fictitious gaze of the figures in the image points out of the space of the image into the physical space of the viewer. In both cases, seeing goes beyond the visible, unfolding into a perceptual-fictional disclosure of the seen. In terms of their expressive quality, the fiction of encounter engendered by the figures in Hill's video is indistinguishable from Sartre's imaginary passer-by, since both generate the feeling of being seen with all its ethical ramifications, its effects of power deprivation, the addressing of the viewer, her unease and so on. Once again, we see that the gaze from an image, like the gaze from a real face, cannot be seen with the intent of determining identity that we bring to inanimate objects.[11]

One of the properties of the images is to both *be* and *have* a sensibly perceptible shape, that is, to be fictitious and at the same time to have a

[11] Even if we concede that tables and chairs can possess a certain appellative force, there remains a difference between seeing objects and imaginary seeing.

phenomenal form that can be perceived. By the same token, it is a property of the face to be both physiognomy and an embodied act of expression. Both therefore exhibit a similar twofoldness and surplus. For this reason alone, dividing the faculty of vision into a physical and a psychic part must necessarily go awry.

The psycho-physical holism of the perceptual practice is mirrored in the artistic process of expression. G. Simmel discussed this in his study of Rembrandt:

> Art in particular represents human appearance in such a way that the duality of the physical and the inner conception – of perception and interpretation, into which the inadequate relationship of the observer to the observed often stretches the observation – vanishes. (Simmel 2013, p. 18)[12]

What Simmel characterises as insufficient is the paradigm of givenness that splits perception into sensible stimulation and mental processing. This apparent duplicity is "in reality and in art one and the same" (ibid., p. 29). We again encounter here the impossibility of denying the duplicity without having presupposed it previously: "Insofar as one spiritualizes sensory seeing, one may render spiritual seeing sensory" (ibid.).[13] Laying claim to such oppositions in order to simultaneously disavow their separation was, as we saw, the crux of Kant's notion of concept and intuition. Simmel comments on this: "if it is true that intuitions without concepts are blind; concepts without intuitions are empty, so it is through their synthesis that unity is created. But this is still a question as to whether or not this unity corresponds to an originally unitary function the separation of which into concept and intuition is not even prefigured in its own structure" (ibid., p. 17).

The proper structure of the relation is its original unity, which is rendered present by the process of expression in art. The holism of seeing is a dialectical mediation of opposites, which preserve their difference within the unity and nevertheless only occur in connection with one another.

[12] The problematic nature of Simmel's ethno-sociological interests compromises his insights into the theory of seeing.

[13] Incidentally, Simmel makes similar points in his aesthetic of the portrait, where the portrait shows "the meaning of its appearance, not the meaning behind its appearance" (Simmel 1995a, p. 321).

2.3 Rembrandt 2: Seeing Made Visible

Rembrandt can help to elucidate seeing as an aesthetic practice in terms of what we have referred to as the iconic, (re)presentational power of showing inherent to perception. I have made the two claims that the history of painting is a history of various styles of seeing, and that both seeing and representing each consist of deictic and aisthetic elements woven together.

Rembrandt's 1646 painting "The Holy Family with Curtain" (Fig. 3) depicts the classic theme from Christian iconography as a contemporary genre piece in an indoor setting. Joseph is seen engaged in his trade while in the foreground the domestic daily life of mother and child is presented in the warm light, the source of which is visible within the image.[14] Remarkably, Rembrandt has embellished the image with a perfectly naturalistic frame and curtain. This measure, a commonplace particularly in Baroque painting, crucially alters the depicted scene. The painter shows us not only

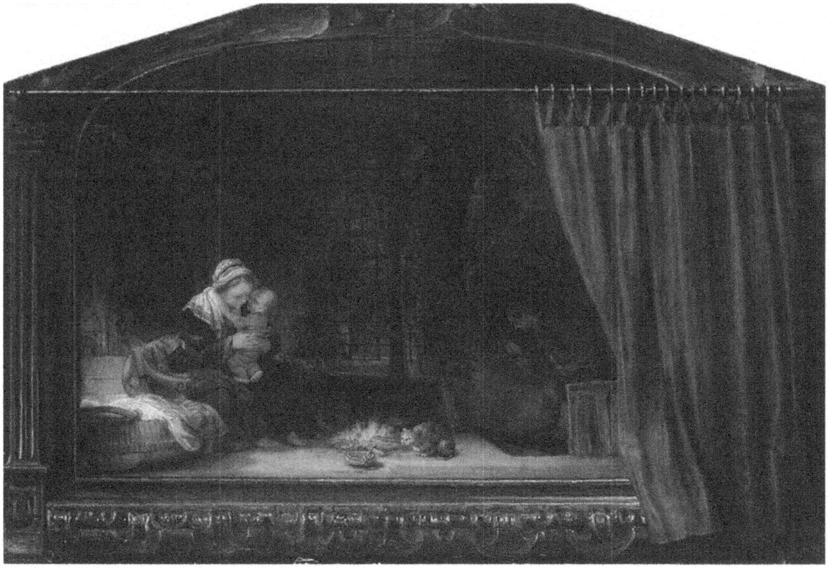

Fig. 3 Rembrandt Harmenszoon van Rijn, *The Holy Family with a Curtain*, 1646, Gemäldegalerie Alte Meister Kassel

[14]For more particulars, see W. Kemp (2003).

what he sees but also *that* he sees and that he *shows* us what he sees. The curtain—originally part of the standard inventory of dominant iconography as an image of religious revelation[15]—not only brings about the effect of a Parrhasius-like trompe-l'oeil.[16] This creates an aesthetic distance, which transforms the image space into a stage and the figures into the protagonists. The frame explicitly reflects the intentional act bracketing and excerpting what is represented. As consciousness for Fichte is a "stage of changing images" (Schulz 1972, p. 330) so the image here is the stage for an imaginary happening.

The representation and what is represented are rendered theatrical in the sense intended by Fried[17] by the way the deictic character of the image itself is shown, thus making explicit the aisthetic character of looking at pictures. The aisthetic act completes the deictic act, the intentional showing something-as-something needs to be realised in the intentional seeing of something-as-something. Hence the claim is justified that the painter makes visible not only something seen but also structures of seeing itself—those structures connected with showing.

3 Cézanne and Kentridge: Seeing-How and Seeing-As

The following comparison of the art of Paul Cézanne and William Kentridge serves to illuminate two aspects: first, I want to demonstrate the foregoing conceptual distinction between syntactic and semantic seeing. Second, this will in turn explain what it means to say that all seeing involves blindness and invisibility, which can, however, be differentiated in their negativity.

In the margins of his "Reflections" on the aesthetic of the sublime in modernism, Jean-François Lyotard makes an interesting remark on the painting of Paul Cézanne. Cézanne's works make us "see what makes us see, and not what is visible" (Lyotard 1988, p. 113). Cézanne, he explains, practices a kind of asceticism that involves freeing the field of perception from prejudices "inscribed even in vision itself" (ibid.). How and with

[15]On the use of this motif since antiquity, see Johann Konrad Eberlein (1982).

[16]Pliny the elder reports in the 35th book of his *Naturalis Historiae* the superlative achievement by which Parrhasius deceived Zeuxis, whose painted grapes only deceived the birds.

[17]On the theatricality of seeing, see the comprehensive study by U. Haß (2005).

which way of seeing and of painting does Cézanne allow us to see the visible world less burdened by prejudice?

Maurice Merleau-Ponty, who makes Cézanne the principal witness of his phenomenology, writes that Cézanne wants to make the "primordial world" (Merleau-Ponty 1993, p. 64) appear by showing the visible prior to its being tailored to perspective. This may indeed be impossible, but it is nevertheless possible that the artistic means at Cézanne's disposal help to explain the preconditions and implications of visual perception that usually remain unconscious.

Both philosophers claim that Cézanne practiced a seeing still uninformed and unbroken by presuppositions, habits and other acts of interpretation, and that Cézanne's painting[18] make visible such pre-predicative perception. Undoubtedly, central perspective can be regarded as a prejudice with which Cézanne breaks by building his images out of colour patches and surfaces, the depth of which is due solely to chromatic rhythms, instead of subordinating the living visual impression to rational ordering principles and a geometrical spatial scheme. He thereby brings out a type of perception that centres entirely on the visible values of colour and form. He admits views from above and below, as well as the moments of blurredness and fragmentation inherent in natural seeing, abstaining from subjecting the seen to a scientific scheme. Such measures can reasonably be regarded as representing a paradigm-shift away from the type of seeing previously dominant in the history of painting. Cézanne's gaze appears to consist in a deliberate looking-away and overlooking that renounces all determinant points of view. A necessary prerequisite of this abstinence is shutting down the gaze that follows cognition.

Cézanne thus makes tangible in exemplary fashion the type of seeing I have called syntactic *seeing-how*. The example displays the different structural determinations of seeing. I claim that *seeing-how* differs from semantic *seeing-as* in that *seeing-how* abstains from attributing identity. In order to demonstrate this, I will compare Cézanne with works by the contemporary artist William Kentridge[19] (*1955). With his shadow pieces (Fig. 7), Kentridge has developed a procedure that gives an illuminating example of semantic seeing.

[18]For good reproductions, see F. Baumann (2000).

[19]For good reproductions, see D. Cameron (1999).

Where Cézanne's original inventiveness consists in refraining from a determination of the object seen, Kentridge, with his silhouettes, practices a *seeing-into*, seeing the figurative into the abstract. Where Cézanne remains inside a way of seeing as a self-purposive act not leading to determination, Kentridge uses it as a means to the end of narrative figuration. While Cézanne abstracts from what he *knows* about the objectively ordered and intersubjectively shared world of perception in order to concentrate on what he *sees*, Kentridge proceeds along the reverse route, discovering contours of possible objects in the non-objective. Both methods are situated within the field of the relative invisible to the extent that both overlooking and seeing-into are more than mere visibility. Cézanne and Kentridge seem to me for this reason to exemplify the interaction between the visible and the invisible in seeing-how and seeing-as.

3.1 Cézanne's Face

Rilke provides a striking description of Cézanne's face in the act of painting: "In unbelievable heightening and at the same time reduced to the most primitive state," in "unseeing stupidity," but at the same time attentive, enduringly wakeful, "eyes uninterrupted by any blink" (Rilke 1983, p. 61). Cézanne stares fixedly at the intended motif. *Quarry at Bibémus* (Fig. 4) brings an image-world of largely undetermined and indeterminable forms in earthen colours into appearance. Several trees can be made out here and there by an inquiring gaze, the blue can also be separated out of the whole and interpreted as sky. But what the many red-brown forms in the fore- and middle-ground signify remains uncertain. This uncertainty is of course partly determined by the motif. A quarry consists of amorphous, indeterminate forms, yet the artist's mimetic intention could have led to a more exact demarcation of the stone blocks for the purpose of greater recognisability. However, although Cézanne's avoidance of sharp outlines corresponds to the edges of the rock formations, a different artistic intention can be surmised.

Cézanne parts with the copy paradigm of the tradition in order to come closer not so much to the object, as to the modalities by which it becomes visible. Admittedly, few works in the Western painting tradition have pursued the ideal of mimesis in the trivial meaning of copying. The artists were primarily seeking after the characteristic. But Cézanne seems to find the characteristic of his subjects mainly in the doing away with replicating the object. The specific appearance of the visible can attain visibility in the

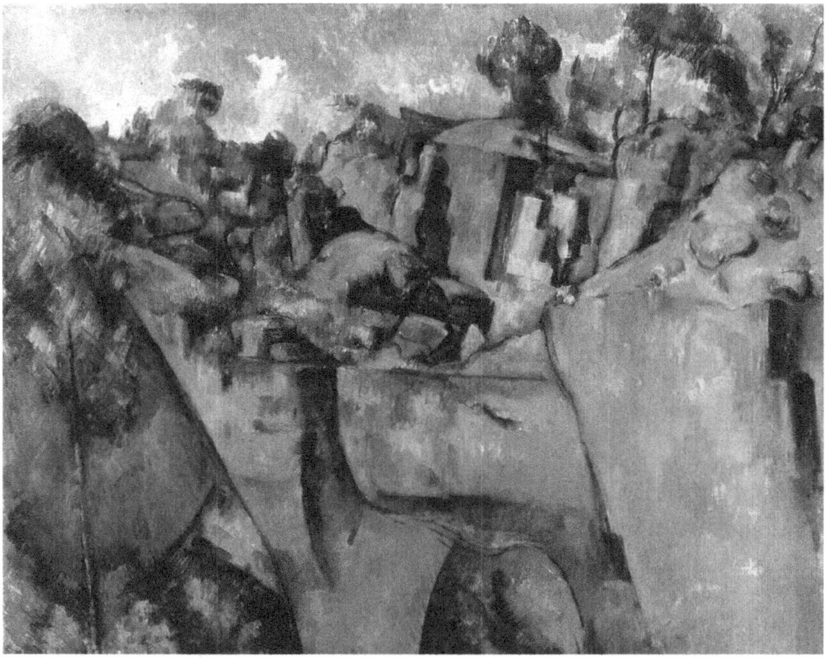

Fig. 4 Paul Cézanne, *Bibémus Quarry*, ca. 1895, Folkwang Museum, Essen

light of its individual situation to the degree to which the painter avoids naturalistic copying. The remarkable thing here is the way the abstract representation of the object still resembles the object seen in nature, despite our expectation to the contrary.[20] This type of resemblance is due not to copying the object but rather to the way the object is presented. Painting is not similar to nature in the sense of a derivative copy. Instead, the emergence of an object in an image is the counterpart of its being visible in nature.

[20]For this reason, the landscape around Aix-en-Provence can appear like a Cézanne to visitors with eyes trained by the paintings. This shows not so much how the gaze can be formed by education but rather demonstrates the curious fact that what Cézanne shows indeed resembles the objects since resemblance cannot rely on mere replicative copying.

It is here that the aspect of freedom from prejudice in seeing plays an important role. Ordinary seeing for the purpose of orientation in the everyday mostly consists in a rapidly executed cursory study on the way to a propositional utterance or an identity judgement of the form "a = b". Cézanne, however, appears to break with epistemic seeing by arresting the process at a point where judgement is not yet possible. His characteristic gaze does not lead to definite determinations. This gaze invests the objects in his paintings with an uncertain status. When the observer approaches the image with an inquiring gaze wanting to know what object is being seen she finds no answer or, at most, only a vague one.

3.2 *Syntactic Seeing and the Non-Propositional*

In the case of the quarry picture, the field of the image is dominated by perpendiculars, frontality and planes. Depth is created almost exclusively by nuances of colour. What is represented floats not only in an ambiguity between different possibilities of determination, but rather in an essential, non-identifiable uncertainty. Cézanne sceptically defers knowledge of possible predications or simply renders it indifferent, thereby representing not only *what* he wants to paint but *how* it presents itself to his sight. In this way, his painting can truly be interpreted as a paradigm shift away from seeing in terms of judgement and instead toward non-epistemic seeing. It is constitutive of the world of intimations and traces of objects, which these images create, that what is being shown remains an open question.

Cézanne's seeing operates syntactically in that it overlooks almost all the ingrained meanings of the seen. It directs itself toward the formal relations of the visible and the quasi-geometrical structure of its visibility. As the syntax of a sentence is based on a general system of rules, so is the visible correspondingly based on general structures made up of colour, form, contour, proportion and so on. The optical presence of objects is organised by values of visibility comparable to sentence structure. Cézanne's forms—his much-quoted cubes, spheres and cones, their lines, reliefs, masses and proportions—are parameters of visibility, not of objects. The concentration of these elementary structures of the visible directs attention to something that remains invisible in the kind of seeing on which mimetic painting is based. Instead of leading to definite utterances about the quiddity of the visible, Cézanne's seeing permits only provisional insights that cannot be translated into propositional statements. What the images show remains alien to all knowledge organised on the basis of judgements. It is as though

Cézanne felt the same amazement as Nietzsche when discovering how little our sentences, with their division into subject and predicate, correspond to what in the world that we try to grasp with them.

Cézanne's gaze is of course logically incapable of entirely escaping the structure of judgement, since even seeing-how is partially dependent on seeing-that. It is however nevertheless a type of non-propositionality, which enables it to focus on syntax, since this focus does not bring the viewer to final judgements on the nature of the object. The simple *that-ness* of the hard-edge optics permits no predication. In other words, it does not lead to *certain* knowledge but instead, and by the same token, to a greater degree of knowledge *by acquaintance*. Instead of judging, as identificatory seeing does, *what* something is, syntactic non-propositional seeing relates to how something shows itself. This involves a productive reduction of the seen to the *how* of its *being-visible for someone seeing*, thus rendering visible something otherwise invisible.

3.3 Abstraction and Concretion

This brings to light a peculiar intermeshing of the general and the particular. Turning away from the will to know and cognise involves an abstraction, which we would expect to bring to view the object in its most general, least individual state. Contrary to this expectation, however, the object represented by Cézanne's reduction of it to a syntactic mode of givenness appears in irreplaceable particularity: it is this object that appears just as it does and not otherwise within the singularity of its spatial relations and its peculiar situatedness. It is a determined indeterminate, not a random form. Its particularity, however, is based on characteristic properties that recur in other specimens of the/its class. It becomes a meaningful singularity when it is seen in a specific context. The image does not show the general scheme of a quarry, but rather a specific view of a particular quarry embedded in specific conditions of light and colour. Cézanne shows not only what is seen, but also the act by which it is seen. In normal seeing, this being seen is covered over by object identification. We recognise a chair as a token of a general class of things by attending neither to its individual particularity nor to the way it is visibly present. Artistic abstraction, however, seeks the genuinely concrete. It is not scientific abstraction, subordinating the particular to the typical. Instead, it blocks the knowledge of the generality of the object in order to render it visible in its particularity.

The concept of style is once again applicable here. A painter's style interlocks the expressive quality of the represented object with the form of representation to make perceptible a characteristic singularity. Cézanne's style of perception unveils the perceived both as incomparable and typical.

3.4 *Seeing as Transformation*

This quality of radically altering the seen makes seeing a meaningful dimension of practice transforming the visible world. Syntactic seeing is a performance that does something with the seen; it presents it in its singularity and typicality, so that it can enter into visibility in an unaccustomed way. The avoidance of predication is not abstraction in the sense of ignoring the individual, but rather, on the contrary, of blocking out the general knowledge of trees, landscapes, rock formations, which allows them to be recognised, in favour of an attentive inspection of things in the incommensurability of their respective situation. The reduction of the seen to these elementary visible characteristics, which permit of no further reduction, shows the autonomy of the visible as the irreducible ineffability of the singular thing.

Rilke's emphasis on the thing found its support in this quality in Cézanne's painting.[21] Rilke's description of Cézanne, however, sometimes makes it seem as though seeing were merely the reception of sensory stimuli.[22] The abstraction away from classificatory seeing is not the innocent eye but rather the conscious effort to become aware of a layer of the visible that is not socially prefigured and thus usually overlooked.

3.5 *How the Visible Becomes a Thing*

Seeing, as an active movement between a viewer and something visible, does not necessarily unfold in time. The image would freeze this movement if

[21] In his "thing" poems, Rilke seeks a form of utterance that is not entirely contained in what is said, i.e. in predication. Cézanne seeks something similar in seeing. See M. Dobbe (1992).

[22] Consider the oft-cited statement that Cézanne sits before nature "like a dog,“ which evokes anew the mistaken notion of a basic ocular activity. Instead, it appears precisely to be an "intelligent eye" that could with Max Imdahl be termed "iconic," a focus on the picture-immanent, simultaneous force of expression due to the action of representation achieved by form, colour and composition. Imdahl's concept of the iconic involves a method of analysing the syntactic order of pictures as a primal element of artistic expression in analogy to Cézanne's concentration on the autonomy of the visible world (Imdahl 1988).

it did not consciously manage to foreground the genetic and transitory aspects of seeing.

The problem of representing movement is familiar to the visual arts. A falling stone remains in a painting an eternally arrested moment unless the treatment of the paint confers on it an optical dynamism.[23] Snapshots in photography petrify movement unless they are *fruitful moments* in the sense intended by Lessing.[24]

In order for the image to not merely be mimetic representation, but rather a real mode of presence of the represented, the object realised must be rendered visible in its temporality. The procedure of syntactic seeing fulfils this requirement. The syntactic construction of the visible world itself possesses a pictorial structure and this structure can only be unveiled by syntactic seeing. By turning away from what an object *is*—for instance, as rock or tree—syntactic seeing turns toward its *modes*, its possible ways of appearing in time. This is the illuminating paradigm shift from mimetic to syntactic seeing or rather from the thing seen to the becoming-thing of the seen.

What images repeat is the becoming of the visible world. The term *realisation* has established itself through statements by Cézanne himself and by research on Cézanne since Kurt Badt (1956). The phenomenal reality of nature is realised in Cézanne's paintings with its own particular temporal dimension. The transference of the seen to an autonomous pictorial composition shows the thing in the temporality of its appearance. The transitory nature of this process is not frozen in the picture. The object is not spatially localised, as indicated by the blurred contours. The picture shows the *seen*, but also its *seenness*, its being seen. In a second move, this seenness is reinforced by the activity of the observer, whose acts of reception actualise the temporality. The visible is organised under the conditions of the image-space such that the phenomenon is as it were generated anew within the surface by means of coloured paint.

This process character of the finished-unfinished has often been observed. Cézanne's paintings make present the natura naturans as opposed to the natura naturata (Imdahl 1981), they generate the object before our eyes (Boehm 1988), "germinating with the countryside" (Merleau-Ponty

[23]On the temporality and experience of the image, see E. Schuermann (2004).

[24]Rodin's sculpture "L'homme qui marche" can be usefully employed to explain the problems of representing movement. See Merleau-Ponty's (2007, p. 272ff.).

1993, p. 67). They show, according to Jonathan Crary, "the understanding that the world can only be engaged with as a process of becoming" (Crary 2001, p. 301). "In Cézanne we engage a motor and sensory attentiveness to the continual emergence and disintegration of constellations of relationships of which the self was a constituent element" (ibid.). The unfinished appearance of the object in the painting creates the genetic impression of a world in the state of being born.

This does not imply that the seen is thereby unstable or erratic.[25] The discovery of the syntax of the visible occasions a coherence in the composition, which lends the objects permanence. Yet the change from the seen to the seenness of things requires a transitory quality in the form of representation that can be accomplished precisely with the syntactic focus on the being-visible of the objects.

3.6 *Kentridge's Media*

The contemporary artist William Kentridge has developed a unique way of making images that involves the interplay of various media. The resulting installations, incorporating film transferred to video, are based on stop motion film shots of charcoal drawings showing different phases of movement and action (Fig. 5).

He begins, for example, with the drawing of a cat. A characteristic form appears on the white sheet of paper, photographed at a specific moment in its development. Additions and subtractions are made to the same drawing and in this way a further stage of a cat in the course of being generated or moving is drawn and photographed. As in cartoon animation, the photographs are run together as a film. Kentridge's animations differ from conventional cartoons in two significant ways. First, not as many individual shots are connected as in a conventional cartoon, which runs through 24 images per second in order to keep the motion fluent. Second, a new drawing is not made for each shot, but instead a single sheet is used for the various phases of the same scene. Every individual phase of the drawn object or episode is photographed. The photographs of the drawings are then run together to produce jumpy, erratic transitions. Almost one week of drawing becomes 40 seconds of a film.

[25] Meyer Schapiro (2004) emphasised for this reason the permanence of the phenomena in Cézanne's paintings.

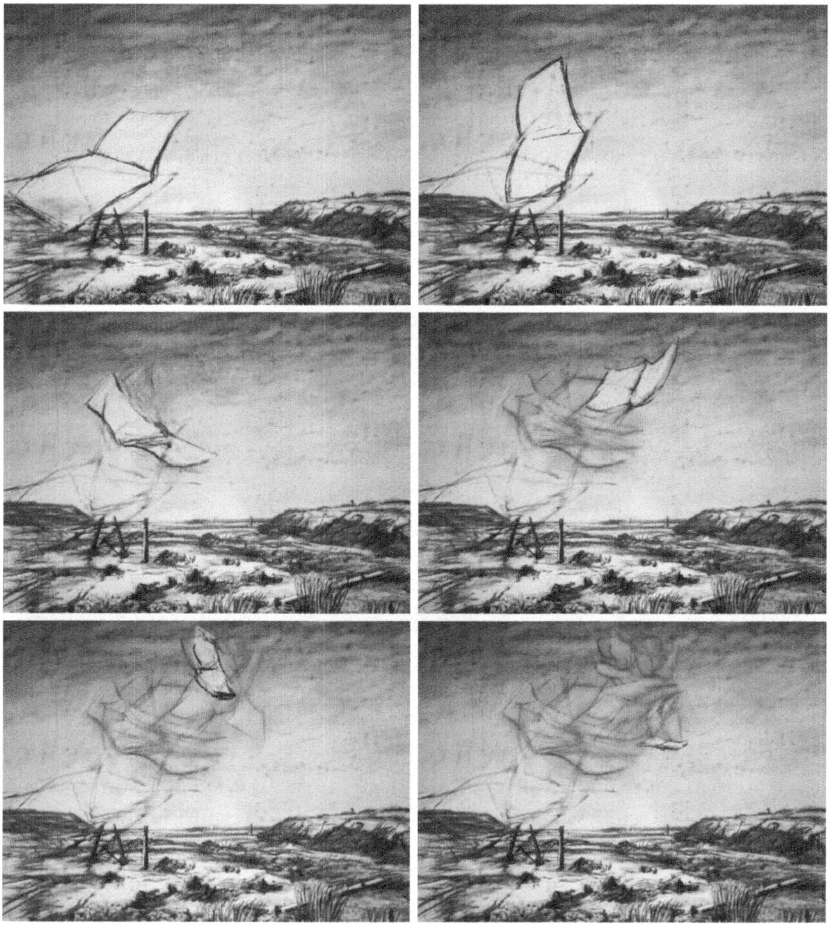

Fig. 5 William Kentridge, stills from the film *Felix in Exile*, 1994, courtesy of the artist (*Source* © William Kentridge)

By means of drawing, photography and film, Kentridge manages to incorporate into the representation the process by which a figure is generated. Figures emerge and pass away on the white surface; situations and scenes are replaced or merge together, are generated out of each other and disappear into each other. The interplay between images gives rise to fragmentary narratives (Fig. 6).

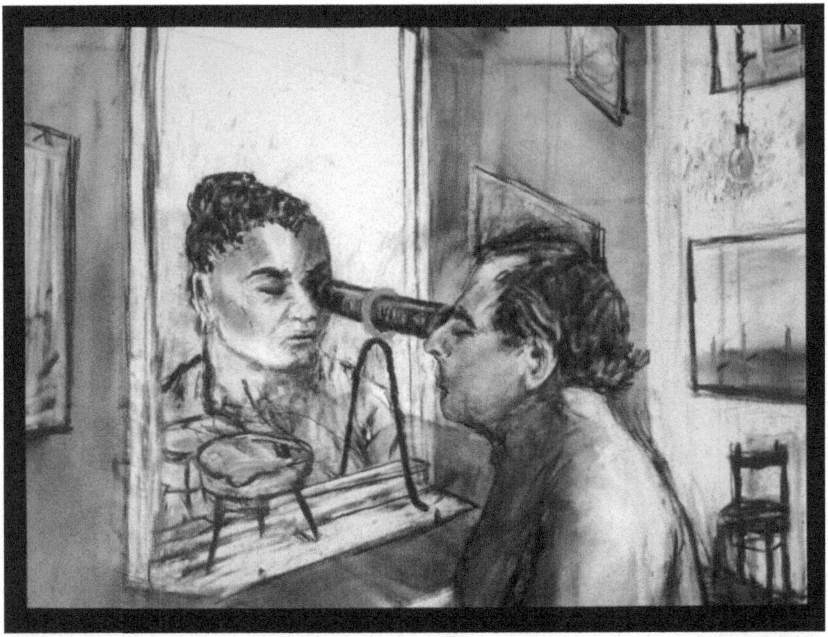

Fig. 6 William Kentridge, still from the film *Felix in Exile*, 1994, courtesy of the artist (*Source* © William Kentridge)

Extinction, erasure, smudging, re-drawing are of special significance. The medium of charcoal permits the repeated softening, alteration and removal of the marks. The blurred marks leave behind visible traces and edges. A vestige of the erased contour remains imperfectly annihilated, the mark is not entirely gone but remains visible as a line, whose genesis can never be reversed. In the palimpsest-like over-layering of images, the upper images render previously visible marks invisible. In this fashion, Kentridge draws "hundreds of instants" (Christov-Bakargiev 2004, p. 5) as the continual occurrence of figures and scenes appearing and disappearing.

The people and happenings mirror facets of a fragmentary narrative. The genetic and alterable presence of the things represented prevents the narrative from being grasped as a stable and fixed order. Instead, a constellation of possible narratives and views emerges and changes before the eyes of the viewer without ever being attachable to an unequivocal story.

Going beyond the aporias of the avant-garde in the twentieth century, Kentridge further develops possibilities of artistic narration with the use of a combination of media, exploring new modes of storytelling that neither classify nor homogenise. Kentridge writes: "I am interested in [...] ambiguity, contradiction, uncompleted gestures and uncertain endings" (Kentridge 1992). His procedure can be more closely described as *enabling* than as *realising* one or more narratives. The hand engaged in drawing and erasing enables lines, forms, figures and pictorial fragments to come into being, while enabling the observer to make images and episodes out of them that are constituted rather by breaks and jumps than by continuity.

The interplay of drawing, photography and video allows manifold moments and points of movement to be joined together to perform anew the movement of the visible world in the act of viewing. A world of images and scenes emerges and vanishes again and again, but never in quite the same way.

3.7 Shadow Figures

So much for Kenridge's artistic procedures. His animations are occasionally varied, when instead of drawings he uses collages of paper silhouettes that he photographs and turns into filmic processions. Black cardboard is torn up to render the contours of figures (Fig. 7).

The fact that the silhouettes are not deliberate, the scissors at most performing a helping role suggests that the results are intended to be equivocal and aleatory. According to Kentridge, the shadow figures result not only from the act of tearing but above all by the posterior activity of seeing by which possible objects are *seen into* the image.

This method originated from a playful experiment with children that the artist has described as follows: "And they made a dog do a somersault, a dinosaur rearing on its hind legs, a monster hiding its head behind its arm. If we had started the other way, this would have been impossible of course. None of them could say or draw what a dog doing a somersault looked like, but all could recognize it as it appeared before them, made by them. It is seeing in – seeing the face in the cloud – that is the basis of the shadow work I have done over the last years" (Kentridge 2004, p. 35).

Kentridge writes about the impossibility of intentionally producing this or that figure. It is however indeed possible to transitively see such figures *into* a torn-out piece of paper. "I take a sheet of paper, I tear it into three or four shapes and place them next to each other" (ibid.). "Objects soon

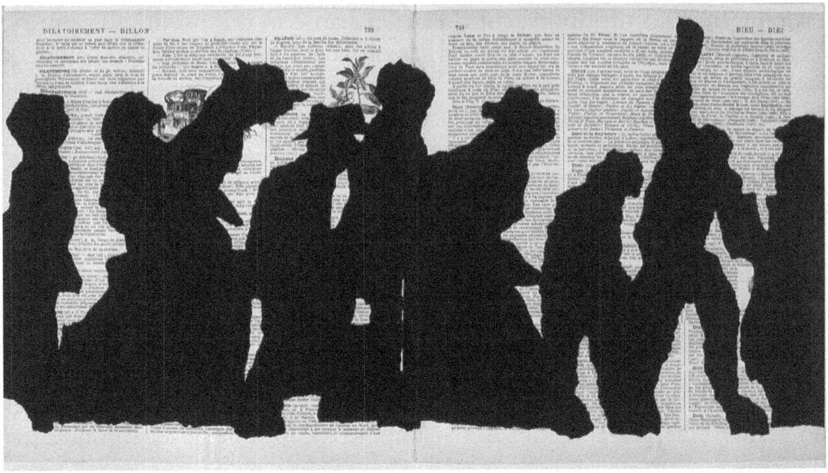

Fig. 7 William Kentridge, *Portage (Carico)*, 2000, Animation (Detail), courtesy of the artist (*Source* © William Kentridge)

start to emerge. In this combination they are a dog, in this combination a man with a stick; I tilt this piece forward and he ages, I lean it back slightly he gains in arrogance. There is a process happening here of the eye leading – of the eye saying, 'Let me show you what I know of the world.' The eye says, 'This awkwardness in the shape in front of you is someone leaning on an uncomfortable hip.' If I had started the other way around, and said, 'Let me make a shadow figure of someone with a limp,' I would be hard pressed to do it. The best I can do is to set in place strategies to allow this image of a limp to emerge. When Rembrandt draws his woman teaching a child to walk, or Picasso does the same, they are not saying, 'I know what this looks like and will carry it out,' they are saying, 'Let me work with a looseness or openness that will allow to emerge what I cannot describe or give instructions for, but I will recognize as it emerges.' This process is not the preserve of artists, talented or gifted people, it is fundamental to what it is to be sighted in the world, an oscillation between openness and recognition" (ibid.). The emphasised passages point out the genetic and transitory make-up of perception and apparition, showing up both as temporal and active occurrences.

3.8 Semantic Seeing and Sense Making

Seeing-into, described by Kentridge as "finding a shape through activity"[26] is a semantic seeing—seeing something amorphous as something figurative. The figure of a limping man cannot be deliberately torn from a piece of paper. The figure can, however, be attained by a way of seeing the piece of paper that reads possible figures into an indefinite form. Seeing-into is an activity involving image-making, figure-making and invention. Leonardo is referring to this sort of seeing when he describes seeing such figures in crumbling or mottled walls (Da Vinci 1802). We also encounter this invisible *surplus of potential* in the visible in the way cloud formations, with their fluctuating, blurred edges, encourage different possible ways of seeing. With his paper tearing, Kentridge explores this dimension of seeing. Both the seeing that leads to the production of the artwork, and the seeing performed later by the viewer can be conceived of as semantic acts. In virtue of their indeterminacy, the paper forms cause the imagination actively to enter into seeing and make its own determinations.

This optical movement is the opposite of Cézanne's. It is not invisible knowledge that is abandoned, but rather an invisible faculty of seeing into things. When we not only see what is presently visible, but also what is potentially discoverable, there is a unification of the actual and the potential. The variety of possible ways of seeing reveals both the temporality of seeing and the visible itself. Seeing clouds is a good example of seeing that embellishes and invents because the clouds' mutability corresponds to the temporal mutability of seeing. By installing the figures in a flux of possibilities, the act of seeing-into realises the temporality of the event.

In contrast to Cézanne, Kentridge's seeing can be qualified as a compositional activity entailing narrative attribution of meaning. It transforms the seen into a meaningful form. It does not desist from recognising things but rather sees the figurative *into* the abstract. A century after Cézanne's seminal "emancipation" of seeing for the abstraction of modern art, an art of the twenty-first century that has left behind the avant-garde opposition between "abstract" and "figurative" can renew exploration of the possibilities of figuration and, with the help of new applications of different artistic means, transpose the seen into the shown.

[26]Artist Lecture as Max-Beckmann-Stiftung Professor at the Frankfurt Städelschule in April, 2005.

The performance character of Kentridge's work is its essential property. If he did not succeed in producing figures and stories emerging and disappearing before our eyes, the work of making semantic meaning would be confined to identificatory determination. So many possibilities of the visible arise and recede that it is impossible to make a definite determination. Polyvalence is thus a property of both Kentridge and Cézanne's work. The individual figure can be determined, accorded predicates, but the way it emerges and changes within the animation as a whole can no more be translated into a propositional statement than can Cézanne's cubes. Individual statements are repeatedly made for fleeting moments but only in order to be repealed straightaway and negated, reinterpreted or obscured, so that the piece as a whole presents itself as inexhaustible.

Once again, it is the object in its particularity that is capable of entering into appearance in this way. Kentridge sees *into* the form the typical attitude of a limping man, which he has derived from the abstract form. Both Cézanne and Kentridge work in opposite ways to bring out the singularity of their objects, taking recourse to typical properties, which, as typical, represent something general. Cézanne makes remarkable details appear in the particularity of its optical situatedness, while Kentridge discloses singularity by means of decisive peculiarities.

3.9 How the Visible Becomes an Image

In both cases, seeing is an activity in the sense of practice, because Cézanne's concentration on the syntax is as productive as Kentridge's semantic seeing, in the sense that their ways of seeing perform an act by which the seen is specifically generated.

Analogous to performing illocutionary acts in practice with a sentence, seeing makes something out of and with the visible. What Kentridge's semantic seeing does with things is an act of meaningful image-making. In and by the act of seeing, forms become figures, figures become images, fragments become stories. The interesting aspect of this process is the openness and mutability with which the individual figures and scenes form themselves into possible images and stories that could have been otherwise. They become something by continually changing and thereby actualising the space of possible free play, the condition of which is precisely that cohabitation of the visible and the invisible which is our subject here. The pictorial dimension of this process resides in the ability of seeing to deploy imagination to extend and anticipate the visible. The visible is a dynamic dispositive that encourages a perception, making the seen world a polyvalent image.

3.10 Seeing as Presentation, Seeing as Performance

The interplay of drawing, photography and film enables the performative dimension of representation to appear. The means of production of the represented is no less the subject in Kentridge than the represented thing itself. The movements of the hand drawing, the erasure[27] and blurring; all these acts leave visible traces of themselves in the representation,[28] forming in equal measure themselves and the thing drawn or its photographic image. The art consists in making the otherwise invisible process of production a manifest dimension of the representation itself. A particular invisibility is suggested when the genesis of the drawing is able to become visible, when a line that was the contour of a figure turns into a horizon line or a vanishing trace of its own being.

Kentridge is no more able than anyone else to make visible the invisible as such. But he can make visible the fact that there is invisibility in interaction with the visible.[29]

In the process, the performance and medial aspects of the representation enter into the image. The particularity of Kentridge's use of his means is the attempt to render perceptible the performance of drawing itself and the way the appearance of the drawing is conditioned by its media. The representational form of the filmed drawing makes present the performance character of what is represented. As a result, the paradoxical simultaneity of mediation and performance production is made visible: the act of seeing-into is a performance that both brings something figural into being and mediates it with the amorphous material that was the starting point. The actions of drawing and blurring are deployed in the medium of animation, such that their traces and their vanishing are part of what is shown. The

[27] In the lecture, Kentridge mentioned in passing that he spent two years searching for special technical means to erase marks completely. Only afterwards did he realise that the traces of the drawing process can be deployed as a particular means of representation.

[28] Didi-Huberman (2002) worked beautifully through this theme using a photograph by Victor Regnau, in which one of the people portrayed remains as a partly erased presence.

[29] This is reminiscent of Foucault's description of artistic fiction: "Therefore, fiction consists not in showing the invisible, but in showing the extent to which the invisibility of the visible is invisible." Quoted in Maurice Blanchot (1987, p. 116).

medium brings itself thus into the thing medially represented instead of transparently conveying what is represented while concealing itself.

By flowing into the representation, the processes of apparition and perception make visible at least some part of the dynamic and mutability of being-visible and being-seen. The genre of animation shows not only objects but also how they became what they are and how they stopped being what they were. The performativity and mediality of the representation make it possible to bring into view the metamorphoses of the visible world, its becoming and its passing away. Here too, the representation is a type of shown seeing. It is by virtue of the artist's gaze that a figure becomes what it is. At the same time, it is the figure with its own power of expression and evocation that offers itself to the artist's gaze as a particular possible way of seeing.

4 The Invisibilities of the Visible

Which systematic consequences can be drawn from these elucidations? Which different modes of invisibility can be distinguished? When seeing, the invisible is present in a different way than when seeing-away-from or seeing-into. If it is true that art as a method of seeing differently reminds us of the existence of the invisible—in the sense not of a correlate to objects but as the condition of possibility of the visible—then it follows that different types of blindness and invisibility should be distinguishable.

The two cases of non-propositional, syntactic seeing are each involved in the invisible in their own way. The semantic adds to the seen, the syntactic conceals part of it. The act of seeing is always penetrated by partial blindness, interwoven with selective exclusion and imaginary amendment. The respective visibilities of seeing correspond to different forms of visibility, because the surplus potential of the visible and the knowledge framework are different things. This is important for gauging vision's capacity for world disclosure because it demonstrates how such disclosure is dependent on the invisible.

Just as showing is based on concealment, so too does sight rely on the partial absence of sight, whether due to intentional oversight or fictional addition. The blindness that consists in not being able to see something concealed when we are at the same time aware of not seeing it, for example because it is behind a curtain, differs fundamentally from the blindness of not seeing *that* we are not seeing. While this type of blindness cannot be grasped analytically, that which Cézanne overlooks is susceptible to description. It is that which cannot be seen, the genuinely invisible, only knowable, framework of the object. Cézanne systematically obfuscates previous knowledge and expectations that would otherwise render the syntax invisible. By contrast, Kentridge fabricates in the visible an image out of the possible. With both artists, it is conspicuous that they are striving for the particular, the characteristic singular. Its particularity composes itself within the style of representation. The style is itself unrepresentable and is the product of the expression of the represented, of the hand of the artist, and of the material in which it shows itself.

In the same way as the gaze becomes invisible when the eyes are focused, and through which, conversely, the eyes as objects become invisible, Cézanne's syntactic seeing transforms an object of knowledge into an object of seeing because his paintings make *what* is being seen vanish behind *how* it is seen. Syntactic seeing loses the overview of the objects to the extent that it gains their particularity. Semantic seeing, on the other hand, dwells in the amphiboly of the formless and the figurative, effectively blinded to the abstraction given in the present in order instead to see a potential form, which, like a double-image, makes the formless invisible.

On the other hand, the gaze that meets other gazes opens itself to an image-like and imagined event fundamentally open for infinite interpretation. The duplicity of being visible and seeing touches another surplus potential, which is made manifest as address and demand. In the gaze, response and interpretation are insolubly joined.

Of a fundamentally different kind is the invisibility of time; the realm of generation and passing away that each of the artists under discussion attempts to make tangible. The otherwise invisible genesis of a Kentridge drawing, as well as the slower progression of images in a film sequence suggest the temporality of both the act of seeing and the thing seen. The kinetic medium of film in Kentridge and Hill makes clear what is achieved in painting by the self-reflection of the representation, or in Cézanne's case, the avoidance of unequivocal rendition of objects. Kentridge's deployment of a variety of techniques makes visible the performance and the media in the work, by maintaining the presence of visible traces of the production process, for example. In Cézanne's work, the mutability of a becoming world taking shape for an observer becomes visible. The genesis and metamorphosis of the visual world are grounded in what is no longer there and what is not yet there, in the absent, the formerly present and anticipation, which are invisibly there in the midst of the visible. The memories of what was formerly present are perceptible vestiges of the representational expression, while their possible interpretations touch the surplus of possibility inherent in the visible that itself is not given sensibly.

This variety within the invisible makes it strictly distinct from the merely non-visible. The invisible is sufficiently there to afford being differentiated according to its various aspects. There remains, however, a common element to them all. The visible and the invisible constitute a relation of mutual actualisation. There is something invisible as an integral element in the processes of seeing and of being visible. The invisible is the foundation required for something to become visible, like a figure against a background and like speech against silence. The visible presupposes the invisible. By bringing out one thing into visibility, attention causes something else to recede, as when shifting between focus and synopsis, detail and context.

Hill's relations between gazes, Cézanne's syntactic seeing and Kentridge's semantic seeing each reveal different possible ways of seeing, but all perform seeing as a practice that affects and represents reality and by which the seen manifests its singularity. All three artists ***make present*** something in the double sense of rendering it visible and making it present in the moment. They actualise the temporality of seeing and of the seen in the process of being formulated as images.

The present examination on the theory of seeing has shown the extent to which seeing is the mode and the object of aesthetic experience. This experience is of course mediated by language and reflection. Nevertheless, the art works are themselves another way of seeing that is, namely, self-reflective and enactive.

References

Alberti, Leon Battista. 1970. *On Painting*. Yale: Yale University Press.

Badt, Kurt. 1956. *Die Kunst Cézannes*. Munich: Prestel-Verlag.

Baumann, Friedrich (ed.). 2000. *Cézanne: Vollendet unvollendet*. Ostfildern: Hatje Cantz.

Blanchot, Maurice. 1987. *The Thought from Outside*. New York: Zone Books.

Bockemühl, Michael. 1985. *Die Wirklichkeit des Bildes: Bildrezeption als Bildproduktion*, 107–134. Stuttgart: Urachhaus.

Boehm, Gottfried. 1973. Die Dialektik der ästhetischen Grenze. *Neue Hefte für Philosophie* 5: 118–138.

Boehm, Gottfried. 1988. *Paul Cézanne: Montagne Sainte-Victoire*. Frankfurt am Main: Insel Verlag.

Cameron, Dan et al. (eds.). 1999. *William Kentridge*. London: Phaidon Press.

Christov-Bakargiev, Carlolyn. 2004. Über Fehlerhaftigkeit als Ressource. In *William Kentridge*, 3–10. Milano: Skira.
Crary, Jonathan. 2001. *Suspensions of Perception: Attention, Spectacle, and Modern Culture*. Cambridge: MIT Press.
Da Vinci, Leonardo. 1802. *A Treatise on Painting*. London: J. Taylor.
Didi-Huberman, Georges. 1992. *Ce que nous voyons, ce qui nous regarde*. Paris: Minuit.
Didi-Huberman, Georges. 2002. Superstition. In *Ordnungen der Sichtbarkeit*, ed. Peter Geimer, 434–440. Frankfurt am Main: Suhrkamp.
Dobbe, Martina. 1992. Wie sollte einer von Farbe sprechen können? *Diagonal: Zeitschrift der Universität-Gesamthochschule Siegen* 2: 74–84.
Eberlein, Johann Konrad. 1982. *Apparitio regis – revelatio veritatis*. Wiesbaden: Reichert.
Elkins, James. 1996. *The Object Stares Back*. New York: Simon & Schuster.
Fried, Micheal. 1980. *Absorption and Theatricality*. Berkeley: University of California Press.
Gamm, Gerhard, and Schuermann, Eva (eds.). 2007. *Das unendliche Kunstwerk*. Berlin: Philo.
Haß, Ulrike. 2005. *Das Drama des Sehens*. Munich: Fink.
Hill, Gary. 1999. *Exhibition Catalogue*. Aarhus: Aarhus Kunstmuseum.
Imdahl, Max. 1981. Cézanne, Braque, Picasso. In *Bildautonomie und Wirklichkeit*, 9–50. Mittenwald: Mäander.
Imdahl, Max. 1988. *Giotto*. Munich: Fink.
Imdahl, Max. 1996. Regie und Struktur in den letzten Gruppenbildnissen von Rembrandt und Frans Hals. In *Zur Kunst der Tradition. Gesammelte Schriften*, Vol. 2, 285.396. Frankfurt am Main: Suhrkamp.
Kemp, Wolfgang. 2003. *Rembrandt: Die Heilige Familie mit dem Vorhang*. Kassel: Museumslandschaft Hessen.
Kentridge, William. 1992. *Drawings for Projection: Four Animated Films*. Johannesburg: Goodman Gallery.
Kentridge, William. 2004. Felix in Exile: Geography of memory. In *William Kentridge*, ed. Carlolyn Christov-Bakargiev, 22–24. Milano: Skira.
Lyotard, Jean-François. 1988. *L'inhumain*. Paris: Galilée.
Menke, Christoph. 1991. *Die Souveränität der Kunst*. Frankfurt am Main: Suhrkamp.
Merleau-Ponty, Maurice. 1993. c. Cézanne's Doubt. In *The Merleau-Ponty Aesthetics Reader: Philosophy and Painting*. Evanston: Northwestern University Press.
Merleau-Ponty, Maurice. 2007. Eye and Mind. In *The Merleau-Ponty Reader*, 351–378. Evanston: Northwestern University Press.
Nancy, Jean-Luc. 2000. *Le regard du Portrait*. Paris: Galilée.
Neumeyer, Alfred. 1964. *Der Blick aus dem Bilde*. Berlin: Gebrüder Mann.

Nietzsche, Friedrich. 1999. On Truth and Lies in a Nonmoral Sense. In *The Birth of Tragedy and Other Writings*, 139–153. Cambridge: Cambridge University Press.

Plessner, Helmuth. 1982. Mit anderen Augen. In *Mit anderen Augen*, 164–181. Stuttgart: Reclam.

Rancière, Jacques. 2007. *The Future of the Image*. London: Verso.

Rilke, Rainer Maria. 1983. *Briefe über Cézanne*. Frankfurt am Main: Insel Verlag.

Salles, Georges. 2001. *Der Blick*. Berlin: Vorwerk 8.

Schapiro, Meyer. 2004. *Paul Cézanne*. New York: Abrams.

Schulz, Walter. 1972. *Philosophie in der veränderten Welt*. Pfullingen: Neske.

Schuermann, Eva. 2004. Zeitlichkeit als Form und Inhalt der ästhetischen Erfahrung. In *Licht und Zeit*, ed. Gernot Böhme and Reinhard Olschanski, 94–104. Munich: Fink.

Simmel, Georg. 1995a. Ästhetik des Porträts. In *Aufsätze und Abhandlungen 1901–1908*, Vol. 1, 321–332. Frankfurt am Main: Suhrkamp.

Simmel, Georg. 1995b. Der Bildrahmen. In *Sämtliche Schriften*, Vol. 7, 101–108. Frankfurt am Main: Suhrkamp.

Simmel, Georg. 2013. *Rembrandt: An Essay in the Philosophy of Art*. London: Routledge.

Snyder, Joel. 2002. Das Bild des Sehens. In *Paradigma Fotografie*, ed. Herta Wolf, 23–59. Frankfurt am Main: Suhrkamp.

Valéry, Paul. 1970. Odds and Ends. In *The Collected Works of Paul Valéry*, Vol. 14, 1–156. Princeton: Princeton University Press.

Index

E. Schuermann, *Seeing as Practice*, Performance Philosophy,
https://doi.org/10.1007/978-3-030-14507-1